T0286413

Technology-Enhanced Healthcare Education

EMERALD STUDIES IN HIGHER EDUCATION, INNOVATION AND TECHNOLOGY

Series Editors: Miltiades D. Lytras and Anna Visvizi

Emerald Studies in Higher Education, Innovation and Technology seeks to provide a multifaceted and interdisciplinary approach to these interconnected topics and invites proposals from all scholars working in these fields. The underlying purpose of this series is to demonstrate how innovations in education, educational technology and teaching can advance research and practice and help us respond to socio-economic changes and challenges.

The series has a broad scope, covering many topics, including but not limited to: learning analytics, open and distributed learning, technology-enhanced learning, digital pedagogies, data mining, virtual and augmented realities, cloud computing, social media, educational robotics, flipped classrooms, active learning, innovation networks and many more.

Interested in publishing in this series? Please contact Miltiades D. Lytras and Anna Visvizi, mlytras@acg.edu and avisvizi@acg.edu.

Published books:

The Future of Innovation and Technology in Education: Policies and Practices for Teaching and Learning Excellence (2018)
Anna Visvizi, Miltiadis D. Lytras and Linda Daniela

Management and Administration of Higher Education Institutions at Times of Change (2019)
Anna Visvizi, Miltiadis D. Lytras and Akila Sarirete

Technology-enhanced Learning and Linguistic Diversity: Strategies and Approaches to Teaching Students in a 2nd or 3rd Language (2020)
Patrick-André Mather

Effective Leadership for Overcoming ICT Challenges in Higher Education: What Faculty, Staff and Administrators Can Do to Thrive Amidst the Chaos (2021)
Antonella Carbonaro and Jennifer Moss Breen

Teaching the EU: Fostering Knowledge and Understanding in the Brexit Age (2021)
Anna Visvizi, Mark Field and Marta Pachocka

Technology-Enhanced Healthcare Education: Transformative Learning for Patient-centric Health

EDITED BY

CRISTINA VAZ DE ALMEIDA
President of Portuguese Health Literacy Society (SPLS), Portugal

And

MILTIADIS D. LYTRAS
Effat College of Engineering, Effat University, Jeddah, Saudi Arabia

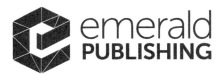

United Kingdom – North America – Japan – India – Malaysia – China

Emerald Publishing Limited
Emerald Publishing, Floor 5, Northspring, 21-23 Wellington Street, Leeds LS1 4DL.

First edition 2024

Editorial matter and selection © 2024 Cristina Vaz de Almeida and Miltiadis D. Lytras.
Individual chapters © 2024 the authors.
Published under exclusive licence by Emerald Publishing Limited.

Reprints and permissions service
Contact: www.copyright.com

British Library Cataloguing in Publication Data
A catalogue record for this book is available from the British Library

ISBN: 978-1-83753-599-6 (Print)
ISBN: 978-1-83753-598-9 (Online)
ISBN: 978-1-83753-600-9 (Epub)

Printed and bound by CPI Group (UK) Ltd, Croydon, CR0 4YY

INVESTOR IN PEOPLE

Contents

List of Figures and Tables

Figures

Tables

List of Charts

About the Editors

Cristina Vaz de Almeida has PhD in Communication Sciences – Health Literacy (ISCSP), President of the Portuguese Society of Health Literacy (SPLS), Researcher ISCSP – CAPP, Director of the Post-Graduation in Health Literacy (ISPA), Editor-in-Chief of the *Journal of Medical Research (JIM)*, Postgraduated in Marketing and in Positive Psychology (ISCSP). Author of books, chapters, and articles in various scientific and technical publications. Also Lecturer and one of the greatest references of Health Literacy in Portugal.

Miltiadis D. Lytras is a Visiting Researcher at Effat University. He is a world-class expert in the fields of cognitive computing, information systems, technology-enabled innovation, social networks, computers in human behaviour, and knowledge management. He is an Expert in Advanced Computer Science and Management, Editor, Lecturer, and Research Consultant, with extensive experience in academia and the business sector in Europe and Asia. He served as the Editor-in-Chief of the *International Journal in Semantic Web and Information Systems*. He has co-edited more than 110 high-impact factor special issues in ISI/Scopus-indexed journals and Co-edited/Authored more than 80 books in international publishers including Elsevier, Emerald, IGI-Global, Springer, etc.

About the Contributors

Sérgio Filipe Silva Abrunheiro is a Specialist Rehabilitation Nurse at the Neurology Service of the Coimbra Hospital and University Center, having started working as a Nurse in 2009. He has been a Member of the Quality and Patient Safety Office since 2022, in the area of Risk Management. He is also a Member of the Health Literacy Group of the Coimbra Hospital and University Center since 2019. He has been a Master in Elderly and Geriatric Health Nursing since 2014 and a Postgraduate in Health Services Management since 2020. He has several published articles in the area of the elderly and health literacy. He collaborated for several years with the Nursing School of Coimbra in teaching classes in the area of Geriatrics. He is a Founding Member of the Portuguese Society for Health Literacy and Secretary of the General Assembly.

Sarah Abdulrahman Alajlan is PharmD, Almaarefa University, Riyadh, Saudi Arabia

Basim S. Alsaywid, Saudi Board of Urology, Pediatric Urology Fellowship (Sydney Children Hospital Network), Master of Medicine (Clinical Epidemiology), Master of Health Profession Education. Pediatric Urologist (Reconstructive), Pediatric Urology Section, Urology Department, King Faisal Specialist Hospital and Research Center, Riyadh, Saudi Arabia. Director, Education and Research Skills Directory, Saudi National Institute of Health, Riyadh, Saudi Arabia

Berta Maria Jesus Augusto, Nurse Manager at the Neurology Service of the Coimbra Hospital and University Center, Specialist in Rehabilitation Nursing, Postgraduate in Health Services Management, Postgraduate in Nursing in Multiple Sclerosis, Nurse in the Regional Coordinating Team of Continuous Care Integrated in the Regional Health Administration of the Center, Coordinator of the institutional literacy group for the safety of nursing health care, and Founding member of the Portuguese Society for Health Literacy, being Vice-Chairman of the General Assembly Board. Participated in several publications and events in the field of continuing care, nursing, and health literacy. Collaborates with the Nursing School of Coimbra, in the postgraduate course in clinical teaching.

José Branco is Medical Doctor at Federal University of Maranhão. Master of Business Administration in Healthcare Executive from Fundação Getúlio Vargas. Specialist in Quality and Patient Safety from Universidade Nova de Lisboa. Patient Safety Executive from Institute for Healthcare Improvement.

Founder of the Brazilian Institute for Patient Safety (IBSP). https://orcid.org/0000-0002-1489-0767

Ana Matilde Cabral is Nurse Responsible for outpatient service at Hospital Beatriz Ângelo. Nurse Specialist in Rehabilitation Nursing. Postgraduation Course in Multiple Sclerosis Nursing. Postgraduation Course in Health Management. Collaboration with Adjunct of the National Program for Diabetes 2016/2017. Participation in the international project 'Diabetes Conversations' as an Expert Trainer in Portugal from 2007 to 2018. Participation, as co-author, in the project 'Pathways of Multiple Sclerosis – Looking, Thinking and Acting in Multiple Sclerosis' and is certified by the International Organization of Multiple Sclerosis Nurses (IOMSN) where four learning guides were enveloped to streamline education sessions in Group.

Ana Marinho Diniz obtained Master's in Nursing with Medical and Surgical specialization. Degree in Educational Sciences. Health Risk Manager at the Patient Safety Office at the Centro Hospitalar Universitário Lisboa Central. Co-coordinator of the Educational and Project Management Department of this office. Collaborates in postgraduate education and clinical supervision of students. Internal audit coordinator. Member of the Scientific Board of the Nursing Journal Enformação. https://orcid.org/0000-0001-9762-9785

Carlos Manuel Santos Fernandes is Quality Manager of the Quality and Patient Safety Office of the Coimbra Hospital and University Center. Coordinator of the Clinical Indicators and Clinical Audits Area of the Quality and Patient Safety Office of the Coimbra Hospital and University Center. Specialist in Community Nursing. Postgraduate in Nursing Information Systems. Postgraduate in Nursing in Multiple Sclerosis. Postgraduate in Health Services Management. Member of the Institutional Group on Literacy for the Safety of Health Care at the Coimbra Hospital and University Center. Participated in several publications and events in the field of health literacy.

Isabel Maria Abreu Rodrigues Fragoeiro has PhD in Mental Health; Coordinating Professor of University of Madeira; President of Health Hight School; Researcher in Center for Research in Technologies and Health Services, Faculty of Medicine, University of Porto (FMUP); and in Laboratório Associado RISE; President of the Scientific Council of the Portuguese Society of Health Literacy; Coordinator of the Regional Observatory of Mental Health of Madeira.

Ana Rita Goes is PhD in Health Psychology and Master in Public Health. Assistant Professor at NOVA National School of Public Health. Her research focuses on health promotion, using the lens of sociobehavioral sciences. Areas of interest include understanding the health needs of vulnerable populations, health literacy, childhood obesity prevention, mental health, behaviour change, and community development, using participatory approaches and a combination of quantitative and qualitative methods. Her recent work includes the assessment of health literacy and organizational health literacy responsiveness and the co-creation of interventions for responsive systems.

Eduardo Manuel de Almeida Leite is an Assistant Professor at University of Madeira with a PhD in Management from University of Trás-os-Montes e Alto Douro. His research focuses on Entrepreneurship, and Management, and he has participated in European-funded projects, collaborating with experts in the field. He is dedicated to teaching courses in Management, Hotel Management, and Entrepreneurship, creating an engaging learning environment. Additionally, he is involved in transnational research networks, coordinates European scientific projects, and holds management positions at University of Madeira. Currently, Vice-President of the Higher School of Technologies and Management, he was an Entrepreneur and Student-Athlete, having been one of the pioneers among former professional soccer players to obtain the title of Doctor in Portugal.

Ana Miguel Ramos Leite is PhD candidate in Political Economy by the Faculty of Economics of the University of Coimbra, ISCTE & ISEG; Master's degree in Public-Private Administration by the Faculty of Law of the University of Coimbra; and Bacherlor's degree in Languages and Publishing Studies by the University of Aveiro.

Isabel Loureiro is Medical Doctor, Specialist in Public Health, Emeritus Professor of Public Health at NOVA University of Lisbon – National School of Public Health. Member of the National Team of the Program Healthy Neighborhoods. Previous President of the Scientific Council of the National School of Public Health, Vice-President of National Health Council, Director of the Department of Health Promotion & Prevention of the NCD at the National Institute of Health and National Coordinator of Health Promotion & Education at Ministry of Education.

Miltiadis D. Lytras is a Visiting Researcher at Effat University. He is a world-class expert in the fields of cognitive computing, information systems, technology-enabled innovation, social networks, computers in human behaviour, and knowledge management. He is an Expert in advanced Computer Science and Management, Editor, Lecturer, and Research Consultant, with extensive experience in academia and the business sector in Europe and Asia. He served as the Editor-in-Chief of the *International Journal in Semantic Web and Information Systems.* He has co-edited more than 110 high-impact factor special issues in ISI/Scopus-indexed journals and Co-edited/Authored more than 80 books in international publishers including Elsevier, Emerald, IGI-Global, Springer, etc.

Andreia De Bem Machado has PhD in Engineering and Knowledge Management. Professor at the Federal Institute of Santa Catarina and Postdoctoral student at the Federal University of Santa Catarina. She is at the National Institute of Educational Studies and Research Anísio Teixeira (Ministry of Education of Brazil). She has been working in the educational field for over 25 years. Currently, her research interests are public policy and political science, innovation, and business management issues: Innovation, education, digital transformation, management, hybrid education, digital technologies, active methodology, knowledge media, entrepreneurship, and knowledge management. She is the Author of numerous articles and book chapters published in national and international journals.

Patricia Martins is Master and Specialist in Community Nursing at ARSLVT to perform functions in the Public Health Unit Arnaldo Sampaio of ACES Arco Ribeirinho. Postgraduate in Health Literacy. Advisor and Supervisor of Clinical Teaching of Specialization Courses and Master's degree in Nursing. Author and Co-author of several publications and oral communications in the field of health literacy. Member of the Board of Directors of the Portuguese Association for the Promotion of Public Health (APPSP).

Dulce Nascimento Do Ó is graduated in Nurse, Specialist in Community Nursing, Master in Public Health, and PhD in Public Health-National School of Public Health (Nova University), with a thesis on Health Literacy and Diabetes. Nurse Coordinator of the Department of studies, projects, and clinical trials and Project Manager at APDP – Portuguese Diabetes Association. Coordinated and participated in national and international projects related with the prevention and treatment of diabetes or other NCDs, health education, health literacy, behaviours change, adherence, and participatory methods in planning, implementation, and evaluation. Co-coordinator of the Diabetes Education Study Group of SPD – Portuguese Diabetes Society.

Karina Pecora performed Bachelor's in Nursing from Centro Universitário São Camilo. Postgraduate in Intensive Care at Centro Universitário São Camilo. Master of Business Administration in Healthcare Executive from Fundação Getúlio Vargas. Specialist in Quality and Patient Safety from Universidade Nova de Lisboa. Founder of the Brazilian Patient Safety Institute (IBSP). https://orcid.org/0000-0002-7871-3321

Raul Marques Pereira is Specialist Physician, Graduate Assistant in General and Family Medicine at the Alto Minho Local Health Unit. He is also Master in Evidence and Decision in Health and Postgraduate in Senior Management of Health Institutions and in Pain Treatment. He is Executive Director of the P5 Digital Medicine Center and Guest Assistant at the School of Medicine of the University of Minho. Created and Coordinates the Chronic Pain Consultation of USF Lethes, the first Pain Consultation in Primary Health Care in Portugal. He founded and coordinates the Pain Study Group of the Portuguese Association of General and Family Medicine.

Susana Ramos obtained Master's in Health Care Infection and Post-graduate in Patient Safety. Nurse Manager and Patient Safety Cordinator at the Centro Hospitalar Universitário de Lisboa Central. Vice-President of Portugal Health Literacy Society. Tutor in the International Course 'Quality in Health and Patient

Safety' at the Escola Nacional de Saúde Pública, Universidade Nova de Lisboa. Co-author of articles and book chapters related to the areas of Risk Management, Patient Safety, Health Literacy, Infection Prevention and Control, Patient Advocacy, and Auditing. https://orcid.org/0000-0003-4043-7955

João Filipe Raposo is Graduated in Medicine (1988) (Medical School of Lisbon University) and PhD in Medicine-Endocrinology (2004) – Nova Medical School (Nova University) with a thesis on Calcium Physiology Mathematical Models. Consultant of Endocrinology (since 2006) at the Portuguese Cancer Institute in Lisbon and at APDP – Portuguese Diabetes Association. Clinical Director of APDP – Diabetes Portugal (since 2008). Guest Professor at Nova Medical School - Public Health, Introduction to Medicine, Diabetology (2006). President of SPD – Portuguese Diabetes Society. Consultant of the World Health Organization for Diabetes and NCD's.

Helena Belchior Rocha, PhD in Social Work, is an Assistant Professor at the Department of Political Science and Public Policy, Sub-Director of the Laboratory of Transversal Skills, and Integrated Researcher at CIES-ISCTE. She has been involved in national and international projects, including two Marie Curie projects, and is the Author of articles, book chapters, and communications in national and international scientific events in the areas of theory and methodology of social services, sustainability, community intervention, ethics, human rights, social policies and welfare, education, and soft skills. Member of the Editorial and Scientific Boards of national and international journals.

Diogo Franco Santos has Masters degree in Medicine at NOVA Medical School|Faculdade de Ciências Médicas, NOVA University Lisbon (2010–2016); General Medical Training at Centro Hospitalar e Universitário de Lisboa Central and Agrupamento de Centros de Saúde (ACeS) de Lisboa Central (2017). General and Family Medicine Specialty Training by Coordenação do Internato de Lisboa e Vale do Tejo – ACeS Lisboa Central, Unidade de Saúde Familiar do Arco (2018–). Postgraduate Student – 'Literacia em Saúde na Prática – Modelos, Estratégias e Intervenção', ISPA – Instituto Universitário, Lisbon (2021).

Ivone Fernandes Santos Silva, Angiologist and Vascular Surgeon, Associate Professor at Instituto de Ciência Abel Salazar Porto, Investigator in Cardiovascular Research Group – UMIB.

Maria José Sousa, ISCTE, Portugal University Professor, with a PhD in Management and a Research Fellow at ISCTE/IUL and CIEO (Algarve University). Currently, her research interests are public policies and political science, innovation, and business management issues. She is a Best Seller Author in ICT and People Management and has Co-authored over 70 articles and book chapters and published in several scientific journals (e.g. *Journal of Business Research*, *UAIS*, *Future Generations Computer Systems*, *Journal of Medical Systems*, *International Journal of Knowledge, Culture and Change Management*, *Knowledge Management*,

WSEAS Transactions on Business and Economics, Information Systems Frontiers, etc.), she has organized and peer-reviewed international conferences. She is also External Expert of COST Association – European Cooperation in Science and Technology.

Cristina Valadas is Director of the Endocrinology Service at Hospital Beatriz Ângelo since its opening in 2012 until the present day. Director of the National Program for Diabetes 2016/2017. Diploma in Therapeutic Education of Chronic Patients from the University of Geneva (2008–2011). Faculty and Founder of the 1st Therapeutic Education Course in Chronic Disease Management; ISPA 2019. PADIS Course – Advanced Training in Leadership, Communication, and Innovation in Health – Lisbon October 2019, taught by AESE. Faculty in the Narrative Medicine Course (Therapeutic Education module) at the Portuguese Catholic University/in partnership with the Faculty of Medicine, Porto.

Preface

A new era of Digital Health has already emerged. Emerging and streamlined technologies challenge the entire lifecycle of health care. In this context, the classical agenda for the discussion of the phenomenon has been enriched with bold, delicate, and emerging topics.

Our book intends to communicate this transformation with an emphasis on health education and the capacity of technology to transform digitally the new generation of technology-enhanced healthcare education. Our basic ideas for the unique value proposition of our multidisciplinary edition are communicated in the next paragraphs.

From the beginning, we have to emphasize that in the centre of our approach and our analysis of the patient. We are very much interested in high-quality patient-centric health care with an emphasis on the utilization of health literacy and the composition of dynamic health and clinical services to move forward the vision of the digital transformation and value-based health care.

The arrival of technologies, such as artificial intelligence metaverse, cloud computing, and many others, strategists, policy-makers, physicians, health literacy experts, healthcare practitioners, computer scientists, psychologists, and social scientists provide a new sophisticated context for the design and implementation of socio-technical medical and clinical health services.

In parallel healthcare education institutions in their quest for a revised, updated, resilient, and robust strategy to reflect on these changes, need to deploy new methodological approaches, adopt innovative methods and vision, and the new generation of healthcare practitioners that will satisfy patients and all the other stakeholders.

In this volume, we bring forward various aspects of this resilient strategy for next-generation digital health and technology-enhanced healthcare delivery:

- Communication of lessons learned, case studies, and experiences from the implementation of digital health projects.
- Coverage of the digital transformation agenda for health education and health care.
- Designing of active and transformative learning strategies for healthcare education.
- Discussion of patient-centric challenges for healthcare education.
- Provision of a novel methodological approach to patient-centric health care.

- Strategizing the use of new technologies for enhanced quality of healthcare education.
- Utilization of health literacy for the delivery of high-quality health care and empowering health professionals, organizations, and communities.

Health research showed that satisfaction with patient centrality are golden rules that health and social organizations should have if they wish to qualitatively increase their services. In this context, the patient's experience means that the humanization of care must be always present and also enhanced with a technological component that utilizes tools and services enabled by artificial intelligence, augmented and virtual reality, and services, such as telemedicine and teleconsultation.

The strategies for the development of services in the areas of health and health education are constantly integrating digital solutions that provide biological, psychological, emotional, individual, and social added value.

The domain of Health Education and Training represents a progressive scientific domain with developments in both knowledge creation and applied practices. It is also related to an interactive connection of health specialists to patients. This is exactly the context of our scientific and methodological contribution through the applied approach we deploy. The development of a volume that captures the latest developments:

- On active and transformative learning for Health Education and Training.
- On Medical Technologies (MedTech) tools that are integrated into the medical practice.
- On instructional design and technology-enhanced learning as an enabler of enhanced quality in Medical Training and Education.
- On policy-making related to the integration of Innovative methodological approaches to patient-centric health training.

The new challenges in Healthcare Education at postgraduate and undergraduate levels require new methodological approaches and transparent integration of active and transformative technology-enhanced learning approaches. From this perspective, our book promotes the best practices and lessons learnt from the current pandemic period and also sets the priorities for the post-COVID-19 eras.

The purpose of the publication is to deliver an innovative edition for health specialists, health literacy specialists, educators, higher education medical experts as well students from medical, nursing, psychological schools, and health management professionals, and to update their knowledge and skills and capabilities with a patient-centric-oriented approach to Health Education.

The volume contributes:

- To the theory and the body of knowledge of the domain of Health Education and Training with novel theoretical approaches and methodological propositions.
- To the practice and the best practices of instructional design of Healthcare Training and Education.

- To the applied knowledge of the domain with key contributions to the integration of academia, industry, and research.
- The edition serves a diverse audience including health specialists and educators in a variety of health sciences.

This edition involves a multidisciplinary team that shares a set of synergies aimed at improving the patient's experience and their satisfaction within health organizations. Teamwork brings together professionals from the fields of engineering, communication sciences, biomedical, patient safety managers, doctors, and nurses.

The methods communicated in this book are based on quantitative and qualitative research, case study, participated and unattended observation, ethnographic studies, and methodologies that use techniques, such as qualitative content analysis, which aims to deepen the participants' feelings, their perceptions and vision of the world and the experiences experienced at the individual and group levels.

This volume also promotes this unique value proposition mix:

- Communication Competences
- Digital Health
- Digital Transformation in Health Education
- Gamification and Health Areas
- Health Education Strategies
- Health Services and Health System
- The Paradigm Shift from the Biomedical Model to a Biopsychosocial Model where emotions work with reason/rational
- The patient experience in the Health System

We thank all the authors who contributed to this book, as well as the EMERALD editors.

May this book open the door to research, to the debate of cases and good practices so that researchers and all those interested in these subjects can improve their performance and knowledge.

Cristina Vaz de Almeida & Miltiades Lytras

Chapter 1

How Digital Health Gives Clues for a Better Health Literacy Patient Experience

Cristina Vaz de Almeida

PhD Communication Sciences and Health Literacy, ISCSP – CAPP, Lisbon, Portugal

Abstract

Humanized digital solutions that provide better access, understanding and use of health services enable better decisions and better patient's experience focused on humanization of care. This translates into better health literacy in the digital area.

Currently health care is inseparable from digital health, and this evidence was highlighted during the COVID-19 pandemic. For this analysis, a cross-sectional study was carried out, with 335 valid answers in a quantitative and qualitative research to evaluate the opinion of the respondents regarding their digital health use and the means used, as well as the perception of emotions generated before and during the pandemic. A qualitative content analysis was also performed on the open question about the future of health.

The results showed a humanization in digital is essential and that it is necessary to prioritize the human relationship and find the meaning of space, communication and proximity of health face-to-face, respecting as differences.

This chapter will also propose the presentation of challenges and results from the application of health literacy on patient empowerment in the health system, based on humanized digital solutions.

Keywords: Health literacy; digital health; communication; health; humanization; patient experience

Technology-Enhanced Healthcare Education:
Transformative Learning for Patient-Centric Health, 1–17
Copyright © 2024 by Cristina Vaz de Almeida
Published under exclusive licence by Emerald Publishing Limited
doi:10.1108/978-1-83753-598-920231001

Introduction

Globally, on 3 February 2023, there have been 754,018,841 confirmed cases of COVID-19, including 6,817,478 deaths, reported to WHO. As of 31 January 2023, a total of 13,168,935,724 vaccine doses have been administered (WHO, 2023).

The pandemic has led to a major imbalance in health systems around the world and the rupture of some worldwide, requiring drastic change in face-to-face care, both due to lack of capacity and to prevent the spread of the disease.

On the other hand, the pandemic required organizations and health systems to quickly move to remote health solutions, given the permanent need for continuity of care for the population (WONCA, 2002).

Digital health has advanced with strength since the beginning of the crisis, as a mechanism for replacing some consultations that allowed instalment solutions of a habit that had to be suddenly changed for both patients and health professionals.

Even patients accustomed to provide online health services crave a frictionless health experience (*Change Healthcare,* 2020). Those who are familiar with digital access still want to have more access to services, schedule *an online consultation,* ask for follow-up/follow-up easily, ask questions with direct answers and pay for the service in one place (Change Healthcare, 2020).

Cacciamani et al. (2020) among the four pillars to face a pandemic, whether telemedicine, tele-education, surgical service and outpatient clinic. But there can be no digital health 'without the effective involvement of health professionals (Thakur & Pathak, 2021), either for telemedicine, tele health, videoconferences or mobile applications for consultations, screenings or follow-up' (Vaz de Almeida, 2020a). However, the sense of space, time and presence were dimensions lost during the pandemic by thousands of people.

Pagoto and Bennett (2013) stress that behavioural scientists are needed to facilitate the translation of digital health innovations, from companies to practical research. We add, however, that behavioural scientists are needed to translate and transform digital health barriers into outcomes for patients. In this transition from the real to a virtual communication skills development is essential to retain the person in this connection and involve them (Ramos, 2020; Rodrigues, 2020) in the process of health and change.

The investment in people, environments and processes was necessary for this change from real/face-to-face to real/virtual to occur. The theoretical principle behind this change is that health and its professionals continue to carry out their mission. It should be ensured that there is reflection and intervention in substitution, maintaining a critical set of the characteristics of a face-to-face environment when moving to a virtual one. In addition, Europe is faced with a high level of low health literacy, where around 50% of people cannot adequately access, understand and use health information (Sørensen et al., 2012; Espanha, Ávila, & Mendes, 2016) and in terms of access to new technologies, there is still part of the population that is very info excluded and therefore leading to inequalities.

Pagoto and Bennett (2013) stress that in terms of dissemination and reach, mobile applications have exceptional potential, much more than traditional interventions and highlight existing scientific limitations, requiring more clinical trials that allow the integration of mobile applications in clinical care, effectively contributing to the clinical and public health impact.

It is also important that in this communication (Kreps, 1988) in distance health, the health professional develops strategies for better retention and memorization, with personalized service and adapted to the age and context of the patient, which stimulate the patient's adhering to health instructions (SNS 24, 2019).

The effort made by health professionals has undergone a greater adaptation to: digital interaction with or without video, use of clearer language and especially with several repetitions. We know that the repetition of information is a technique of health literacy (Almeida et al., 2020) that promotes memorization.

Digital health solutions can provoke a revolution in the way people access services, promote their health and well-being (Vaz de Almeida, 2020a), achieving higher health standards (WHO, 2020). There are some services that can be performed using only the phone as can be seen in Chart 1.1.

Ferreira et al. (2012) analyzed, in an observational study, prospective in a sample of 453 patients included in the INR telemonitoring system (*International Normalized Ratio*), from 2006 to the end of November 2010, the efficacy and safety of a telemonitoring system of patients undergoing anticoagulant therapy. Ferreira et al. (2012) consider that technology is at the forefront of healthcare and self-monitoring projects over the phone, mobile phone or internet are important, and that the telemonitoring system is safe and effective in the remote control of INR analysis.

For Medeiros et al. (2020) telemedicine is a logistics solution for remote medical care, allowing the disseminating of guidelines and ensuring greater accessibility of the patient to the health service. Medeiros et al. (2020) developed a descriptive study of a qualitative nature, through a report of telemedicine experience with care to patients and collaborators of a oncohematological centre, to mitigate the transmission of COVID-19. It is concluded that the strategies

Chart 1.1. Services Performed With Telephone Use.

1. Visits established/scheduled by telephone for meeting between patient and health professional

2. Virtual *check-ins: fast check-in* (five minutes average) with patients via phone or other device, to decide if a visit to the health unit or home is required

3. Review of images submitted by patients. These can record videos and/or images and send it to the healthcare professional (store and forward)

4. Electronic visits: visit to the asynchronous office between patient and health professional through a patient portal or by email. These requests are then answered asynchronously

5. Remote monitoring: physiological data, through parameters with medical devices

Sources: Own elaboration based on Almeida et al. (2020) and Vaz de Almeida (2020a).

that facilitate the doctor–patient contact in the distance modality, especially in a scenario, are important measures to ensure the perpetuation of care to cancer patients; monitoring of oncologic complaints; as well as a better management of hospitalization.

In the case of employees, Medeiros et al. (2020) emphasize that this strategy allowed a better organization of scales, according to the need for confinement, and the possibility of contacting employees routinely, facilitating the early detection of possible symptomatic cases within the clinical staff. They conclude that the association of this distance care, through an institutional platform that has distance service for employees, can allow early decision-making and with lower negative repercussions on local transmissibility (Medeiros et al., 2020).

Palmeira et al. (2020) evaluate the experience of nursing telemonitoring of overweight women, through a descriptive study, with a qualitative approach, conducted at the outpatient service in obesity, in Salvador-Bahia, Brazil, with 42 overweight women. Among the results obtained through testimonials, the central category 'increasing self-care awareness' emerged, which was represented by three thematic categories: (1) experiencing frequent and interactive feedback with the nurse for weight control; (2) improving self-care; and (3) feeling satisfaction with the results achieved. The results showed that educational activities through tele-nursing, from a dialogical perspective, contribute to enhance self-care.

Methodology

This study is quantitative and qualitative and was based on a questionnaire survey, disseminated (online) by the social networks and the networks of each researcher through LinkedIn, Facebook, *WhatsApp and by email*, and an analysis of content of the open response. *LinkedIn* is a professional-run network and *Facebook is the largest online* social network, bringing together 2.45 billion monthly active users (Clement, 2019) and almost all *social media users are* on this network (Influencer Marketing Hub, 2019).

The questionnaire consists of 19 questions, of which 18 closed with a yes or no answer required to continue the questionnaire, and an open question of non-compulsory answer (p. 19) *about what my opinion will be about what the future in health will look like in Portugal?*

The aim of the questionnaire was to know the respondents' opinion related to their situation regarding digital health and the means used, as well as the perception of emotions generated before and during the pandemic.

The questions sought to ask whether people consider health important to themselves; new health technologies such as teleconsultations (Ferreira, 2018), if they have ever accessed this type of health service and feel comfortable having/receiving visits/consultations through digital means are considered effective and important.

From the perspective of health literacy and the size of access, the person was asked whether they can easily access digital platforms linked to health (e.g. through SNS 24, My SNS, teleconsultation with their Hospital or *Health Unit, call center appointment*).

Regarding the relationship with the health professional, it was asked whether they prefer to be attended in person by physicians, nurses and other health professionals, and also feel accompanied by health professionals and, in this health relationship, whether the manifestation of affection (therapeutic) is an important factor.

In the psychological and affective domain, questions were asked about the perception of loneliness in the face of a pandemic and about well-being. Regarding the dimension of understanding, it was asked whether it is easy to understand at first what the health professional tells him.

On the communicative and relational aspects, it was questioned whether health professionals should be more careful in how they communicate with people when working through digital platforms (e.g., a clear and accessible language), support the understanding of health content, be positive and support the user/patient and whether there is digital health without affections and emotions. To evaluate the attitude and behaviour of the core of the person's relationships in relation to health through digital, family and friends were asked whether family and friends are people interested in digital health (at a distance).

The Digit2Demic questionnaire survey was applied from 15 September to 21 October 2020.

To clarify more deeply some of the answers obtained a new questionnaire was carried out with nine ($n = 9$) brief answer questions and disseminated to the geographical areas and institutions that had the greatest participation: geographical area of Greater Lisbon (Setúbal) and geographic area of Coimbra. Within these areas, one of the researchers disseminated with her network of contacts aces Arco Ribeirinho and the network of personal contacts, and another researcher dissected at the University Hospital Center of Coimbra (CHUC) between 5 and 25 November 2020.

This second questionnaire served to deepen a set of questions related to the importance of follow-up and that professional the respondent would choose in this distance health follow-up; as well as what it considers important to have a relationship in health through digital means; the importance of affections and what are the consequences if it does not exist and felt greater loneliness during the pandemic. A solution was also requested for what can be done.

In the evaluation of the answers to the open question, a digital analysis of the respondents' sentiment was performed and a cloudwording was evaluated using *the digital platforms DriveWordCloud, TagCrowd* and *SEOscout.* Thus, it was possible to highlight not only the recurrence of each theme addressed in the answers, but also the repetition of certain words and their contextualization. The strengths and weaknesses were also determined and assessing a global feeling to the result of the responses.

Findings

The Digit2Demic online questionnaire survey obtained 335 valid responses of which most respondents are female (80%) and 20% of whom were male.

As for its geographical location, the majority of respondents are from Coimbra (51.3%), Lisbon (18%) and Barreiro (9%), and have a high educational level (93.4%), with 66% of people licensed and 27.4% with a master's or doctorate.

Most people (98%) answered that professionals should be more careful in the way they communicate and how they do it, reinforcing what the other literature says about the importance of people staying connected and with a social relationship.

Regarding the analysis of results, carried out with SPSS v25, we obtained confirmation that health is important for almost 100% of respondents, before and during the pandemic, having increased slightly in the response 'during the pandemic' from 98.81% to 99.4%. The second deepening questionnaire that was made and disseminated in the region of Setúbal and Coimbra (CHUC) resulted in the idea that it is necessary to work on the understanding and acceptance of these alternative solutions in the first place, to reduce the stigma that only face-to-face consultations give results.

It was also evidenced that digital health must have environmental and psychological conditions to be able to function in the best way, namely the sense of space, communication and affections, which are brought from the relationship in face-to-face health, while respecting their differences.

The vast majority consider new technologies in health important, from 72% (before the pandemic) to 88.3% during the pandemic, although the increase in access to teleconsultation between the period before the pandemic and during the pandemic was only 9%, from 37% to 46% of people who resorted to teleconsultation services. On the other hand, there has been an increase of almost 30% in the comfort of people surveyed to receive consultations through digital means (49–75%) although there are still 25% who do not feel comfortable with this system during the pandemic.

Respondents also consider that communication in health made through video conferencing (with image and sound) became more effective during the pandemic (43.5–58.2%).

In relation to the preference for face-to-face care by physicians, it decreased from 94.3% to 74%, respectively, before and during the pandemic. There are 26% who reported not preferring face-to-face care by physicians during the pandemic (6–26% of negative response). Also, preference for face-to-face care by nurses decreased from 93% to 76%. The number of people surveyed who do not prefer to be attended in person by nurses increased from 7% to 24%, and the variation was similar in relation to the previous question (care by physicians), and in physicians the variation is 20% and in nurses 17%.

The respondents prefer the face-to-face relationship with the nurse if we compared answers 2 and 3. However, *they consider it important to follow up regularly, in which teleconsultation may be an alternative in the impossibility of face-to-face follow-up or to facilitate the contact of patients with professionals.*

Regarding what they consider most important in this distance follow-up by the health professional, the response to the second deepening questionnaire focused mainly on the profile of the health professional, the confidence generated in this relationship, their competence, and therefore their knowledge, abilities and attributes (Tench & Konczos, 2013).

As for the attributes of the professional, in this follow-up is better, he/she must have empathy, availability and interest in patients. As for the size of their skills, the health professional is required to be able to *know the health situation and problems, not to always ask the same questions*; keep his word and call *when he says he will call.*

Solidarity was also raised as well as a repeated concern and guarantee in data protection. When asked if they prefer to be cared for by both professions (doctors and nurses) in person, there is a decrease from 95% to 74%, equivalent to less than 21% of people who prefer to be attended in person and 26% who respond that they do not prefer face-to-face care (p. 4). The reasons relate to their fear of face-to-face contact being able to spread the disease.

There is a split almost half over those who feel and those who do not feel accompanied by health professionals (question 5). There are 49% of people who report that they do not feel accompanied by health professionals during the pandemic versus 85% who felt accompanied before the pandemic.

Affection is important in the health ratio to 96% before the pandemic and 92% during the pandemic. There was a slight increase in those who consider that affection is not important in the health relationship, having gone from 5% to 7% (2% variation). This relationship of affection is important *especially for the construction of a bond with the user.*

In the questionnaire and deepening on the issues of the existence of affection in the context of the relationship in health through digital, the respondents reveal that the lack of affection by digital health services has implications for trust, omission of situation, and problems and respect. The respondents of this deepening questionnaire report that there is mistrust, inhibition, lack of will and security with these consultations, non-compliance with the indications given by the professional, have no desire to expose the doubts and problems you face or even omit problems.

The lack of demonstration of affection and proximity through digital was, in most cases, affirmed by all respondents, *and that this lack of affection in the therapeutic relationship leads to and aggravates isolation, loneliness, depression, especially of the older population.*

In the dimension of health literacy, relative to the immediate understanding 'at first' of what the health professional says decreased from 93% to 79%, a variation of 14%. For 21% it is difficult to understand the first-time health professional during the pandemic, a growth of 13% when asked about their perception before the pandemic.

There are still 31% of respondents who do not know how to easily access digital platforms, although they have decreased that number from 37% before the pandemic to 31% during the pandemic. We can combine this answer with question 13, which reveals 9% of people who had increased access to teleconsultation during the pandemic.

Question 9 shows an increase in the perception of loneliness among respondents, from 41% before the pandemic to 83% during the pandemic, a growth of 40%. Only 17% report that they have no perception of loneliness.

As a solution pointed out, some of the respondents report that a strategy to reinforce the accessibility and participation of the person in his health would be useful in the *creation and reinforcement of multidisciplinary teams that can perform home visits (with the necessary care), or through video calls.* This solution would also benefit the feeling *of loneliness and anxiety generated by distancing from face-to-face contact.*

When we go deeper into the question of whether there is more loneliness during the pandemic and what could be done to combat loneliness, the total number of answers confirmed that *there is loneliness, especially among the elderly.* But there are strategies (European Commission, 2020a)to keep people in touch and accompanied by: (1) the maintenance of social activities in smaller groups, and for people who are more isolated, regular visits; (2) maintain family and social contact through digital means on a regular basis or, in the case of the elderly, proximity network through state security forces, such as national guards, social support teams of municipal councils and parish councils, local associations and volunteering; or (3) a helpline that signals situations of loneliness to a local home support team with regular visits that promote stimulating occupational activities, allowing digital interaction with other people. It was also proposed the continuity of some outdoor activities, with reduced groups of people and fixed, as well as cultural activities and television programs directed to the well-being.

We verified in fact that the perception of well-being decreased from 91.94% (before the pandemic) to 64% (during the pandemic), corresponding to a variation of 27% of the total respondents. There are also 36% who say they do not feel well-being frequently during the pandemic period.

When asked to answer the second deepening questionnaire, to know what is most important to the person, so that there is a relationship in health through digital means, the answers were based on trust, credibility, qualifications guaranteed, skills, sympathy, the protection of patient data and the professional secrecy that is necessary for the health professional to have.

The pandemic process confirmed that teleconsultation does not replace face-to-face consultation, although the 'no' response was lowered compared to the previous one (94.3%) during the pandemic (88%). Only 12% positively stated that the teleconsultation replaces the face-to-face consultation.

The large percentage of responses states (96.4% before the pandemic to 98%) that professionals should be more careful in how they communicate when working through digital platforms. Family and friends become more interested in digital health, from 22% to 46.5%. However, more than 50% (53.4%) remain uninterested in digital health.

And the Future of Health?

A qualitative content analysis of the 197 answers to the open question was performed.

In the general analysis of the results, there was a slightly positive feeling (56%).

The answers are very focused on the reality experienced between March 2020 and the date of the questionnaire survey (March to September 2020) and respondents demonstrate through the answer to the open question (p. 19) a difficulty in assessing the future reality.

Proceeding to an analysis through *the word cloud*, it is the concept of 'technology' that emerges, with 39 repetitions for 'digital', 18 for 'technology' and 17 for 'teleconsultation'. Also the word 'face-to-face' is evidenced with 22 repetitions.

Among the positive points that respondents highlight regarding their vision for the future of health are the following: (1) the future of health involves access to more digital health; (2) this new access to health can be an effective response to lower costs in the NHS; (3) digital access may also be the answer to rapid diagnoses of specific and less serious diseases, reducing unnecessary travel to emergency services (e.g.); (4) contagious diseases are also more controlled; (5) patients with motor or dislocation difficulties may be monitored more comfortably for themselves; and (6) it can lead to an increase in home support to the elderly and even an increase in unconventional therapies, such as osteopathy, among others.

On the other hand, a set of responses with a negative view of the future of health was also called by respondents. Thus, they consider that (1) the distance between patient and health professional can lead to a decrease in confidence in traditional health care; (2) digital media cannot fully replace face-to-face consultation with a social issue of quality in medical follow-up; (3) massive digitization of health can cause greater inequities, with a forced removal of people with lower digital literacy, especially the elderly, away from urban centres, and lower social classes, to the detriment of a higher-income population, more educational and urban level, making quality health more accessible to those who have more money; (4) the elderly population of Portugal, which has been increasing over the years, may become even more isolated and with greater difficulty in monitoring new technologies; (5) the pandemic represented delays in surgeries, cancellation of consultations, difficult access to emergencies, etc., situations that cannot be replaced by digital reality; (6) the ease of digital technologies can give a false sense of savings, causing global investment in the NHS to degrade further, impacting the overall quality of the public health system in Portugal; and (7) it can lead to greater misinformation through an autonomous research of information on symptoms and pathologies with human risks, due to self-diagnosis and self-medication that may have consequences for the health of the population (Chart 1.2).

Evaluating the answers to the second deepening questionnaire, the question of the importance of the health organization and its professionals contributed to the non-existence of a *feeling of abandonment and the user's disinterest in their health*. To meet this need, some of the respondents report that there is indeed more *solitude, but there is an open field that can supply it, through the use of the various digital tools that can establish some contact.*

Regarding the follow-up of the patient through a professional who can be regular in the contacts at a distance, the general opinion was that *the follow-up by the same professional allows a closer relationship and the fact that it is the same professional, allows to give a feeling of stability to the patient.*

Also, in this follow-up of the same professional, the opinion of the respondents emphasizes *that the professional should already know the user previously, who has previously had a face-to-face contact.*

The importance of patient follow-up over the time of the pandemic was clear. More than being face-to-face or digital, *the lack of follow-up of people with*

Chart 1.2. What Is My Opinion on What the Future in Health Will Be Like in Portugal?

Positive Self-perception	Negative Self-perception	Critical Self-perception
Greater follow-up through teleconsultations Best national health service	With various shortcomings and increasingly evidencing social asymmetries, if nothing is done to counteract it I believe that people without access to digital media and with greater difficulty using these means will have difficulty accessing health care in pandemic situations and may complicate their clinical picture Increasing difficulties in accessing them	I think we're going to go back to the same thing
Digital health is inevitable, we must provide professionals with communication skills	It is very compromised if there is no constant adaptation to the new media	Just like it was
It goes fast, but it also goes to a lot of people. On teleconsultations, they will favour the attendance of a greater number of people in distant places	Despite digital media, there is currently a brutal lack of accessibility in my perception, which is explained mainly by the limitations of the health institutions themselves	I believe that health in Portugal will be severely conditioned over the coming months/years
Greater proximity through digital channels, for cases where it is not necessary to be in person	Progressive degradation of human contact with the corresponding unaccountability of the responsible entities devaluation of health agents (doctors, nurses and assistants)	If we raise awareness of the population, health could have a good future Without neglecting the population that does not have access to these platforms

Chart 1.2. (*Continued*)

Positive Self-perception	Negative Self-perception	Critical Self-perception
The use of digital platforms should be considered whenever possible and which do not compromise the effectiveness of consultations and diagnosis, even after the pandemic	I predict a dark future Less empathy It is shameful that you do not die of COVID-19 and die of lack of health care provided Reducing adequate and effective assistance to an increasingly elderly population with high poverty rates More and more sick people without access to consultations	I believe that we will move from face-to-face approach to hybrid methodology, in which, according to the needs and circumstances, digital media can be used whenever possible
It is a path of no return, due to the speed in which it is possible to reach more people	Chaotic. I'd like you to invest in the NHS Concerned about the lack of professionals in much needed areas Very unequal between public and private and rich and poor There is a constant disinvestment in the area of health and the future of the NHS (SNS) is not guessed sympathetic	It is essential to adapt resources for a true centrality in the citizen and an honest bet on the training of professionals to meet the health needs of the population, in a different but integrated dynamic
If responsible institutions and health professionals become aware that technologies should be a complement and not a substitute for human contact, we have everything to make the future of health in Portugal bright	The future of health must be rethought. If, during the pandemic, we forget all the other aspects of health, leaving primary health care and the prevention of diseases other than COVID-19 to the background, then we are further away from the health care of excellence to which we contribute	In my opinion, it will be a mixture between face-to-face and telehealth With various service formats, promoting technology to accompany your users, teleconsultation, telephone, email and face-to-face

Source: Own elaboration.

chronic diseases can aggravate their health status, which can result in consequences that could be avoided, and that will affect the quality of life of the user.

Especially the elderly patient needs further follow-up, and also because most are not familiar with the new technologies, although the telephone call is considered the easiest and most productive (even with video call) there should be a redoubled care by the health professional. The opinions given in the second deepening questionnaire reflect *that it is important to clarify all doubts and demystify the user's concerns.*

Discussion

Digital health brings positive and negative challenges for the population. In the relationship in distance health, the requirements of trust, credibility, friendliness, competencies, data protection and confidentiality are highlighted by the respondents as indispensable factors in maintaining the therapeutic relationship of health.

New technologies become more important day-to-day for all people, even for the most info excluded persons, as they have been an imperative substitute for consultations and face-to-face follow-up either in primary care or in hospital.

As in the results of the Digit2Demic questionnaire survey, through the qualitative analysis of the open question, the maintenance of the patient, over time, with the same professional or the same team generates greater safety, satisfaction and empowerment of the patient mainly through the sharing of data with a permanent staff of nurses (Nissen & Lindhardt, 2017).

Regarding the criticisms made by the respondents, to increase access to the service and information, the understanding of its content and the use of this information digitally, health professionals have to meet the principles of health literacy (Vaz de Almeida, 2020b).

Lobban et al. (2020), in a mixed study, evaluate an online supported self-management toolkit *for family* members of people with psychosis or bipolar experiences and the barriers felt by family members as well as professionals, highlighting: (1) the difficulties in giving priority to the patient's relatives; (2) the technical difficulties of using the tool used (REACT); (3) poor interoperability with information technology systems; (4) lack of access to mobile technologies; (5) lack of training in information technologies; (6) a population limited in technology, which can lead to low levels of use; (7) staff's fears of managing online risks; (8) and uncertainty surrounding the long-term availability of the REACT tool; (9) cost-effectiveness with potential impact on workload; and (10) the possibility of inequalities in access to health care.

Reinforcing the results of Digi2Demic, Medeiros et al. (2020), Jandoo (2020), and Reid Chassiakos et al. (2016) list the benefits felt, which positively promote health at a distance: (1) it is the easy accessibility of patients to their health professionals; (2) the exemption from the need to travel to the health organization, influencing the economic gains; (3) better time management with stricter programming of the agenda of both; (4) the ease of communicating with the health professional and *vice versa*, as well as the patient to ask questions regarding his illness or health status; (5) to prevent the spread of the disease (pandemic); (6) flexibility and ease of telephone access; (7) the importance of knowing the health professional in advance and the person always being accompanied by the same professionals; (8) the regularity of contact; (9) the possibility of strengthening patient education more incisively; and (10) the transmission of a sense of safety to patients, through the continuity of formal and informal contact.

The pandemic has brought the ability of health organizations to make structuring decisions (Brach et al, 2012), such as changing almost radically the standard of face-to-face consultation for distance consultations. In this process, both the professional and the patient had to adjust to innovative practices. The focus should always be on the person. Although digital health cannot be replaced by face-to-face health, as highlighted in the questionnaire survey, a path is opened through digital platforms to use some relational and communicative strategies of face-to-face consultation, based on the principles and dimensions of health literacy. Thus, the goal is to deal with people's health, prevent the disease (especially psychological ones) and promote health and well-being so that they can access health services and information, understand the message, evaluate and use the information to take care of their health.

Technology does not make the change itself without having well-prepared health professionals who should also have the preparation and training by people specialized in psychology (Pagoto & Bennett, 2013) and in communication and health literacy (Vaz de Almeida, 2019).

The involvement of the patient in the process, so that he makes correct and competent decisions for their lives or who depends on them, is reinforced with the development and application of a good communicative, relational process that puts the person at the centre. This communicative process, as noted in the second questionnaire, is important so that the user does *not feel that because it is a consultation/follow-up at a distance there is more coldness in the way it is treated.* Meeting the results of the Digit2Demic questionnaire survey, also Van Lieshout et al. (2020) highlight that the implementation of digital health technologies (European Commission, 2020b, c, d) does not yet reconcile the importance of interpersonal relationships with conventional implementation strategies. The authors (Van Lieshout et al., 2020) recognize the centrality of relationships, so they suggest that implementation teams can better plan the adaptations needed for new technologies to work for both patients and healthcare professionals who run a remote monitoring program to build relationships. As a final result, these relationships and other sources of activity can lead to a technological reach of the expansion of remote health activities (Van Lieshout et al., 2020).

Fear and anxiety were also manifested in the responses to Digi2Demic, confirming what the other researchers who specifically addressed the psychological effects of the pandemic analyzed (Jiang et al., 2020; Serafini et al., 2020; Viana & Lira, 2020; Waller, 2020; Zhang et al., 2020).

In general, we found that well-being decreases among people associated not only with health issues, such as loneliness and isolation, but also with the lack of social connection.

Regarding the limitations of the study, we highlight two: (1) the fact that it was a convenience sample; and (2) there may also have been a bias for the majority of these respondents to have this higher academic profile (bachelor's degree, masters and doctorates), since the own networks of each of the researchers and the platforms used to disseminate the *survey by online questionnaire* were mainly used, it was mainly *LinkedIn*. We therefore verified the quality of the sample in a geographical concentration of respondents with a high level of education.

Conclusion

The results of this research show that people in the field of digital health want to find a sense of space, communication and proximity that occurs in face-to-face health, while respecting the differences that exist in these two dimensions of health. Most of the answers focused on the statement about the future: 'Very digital. Increasingly digital' with a positive and negative issue.

Digital should, on the one hand, be a facilitating and even priority means in monitoring the health of some patients, with a particular focus on chronic diseases. However, it cannot replace the physical with questions of diagnosis and the relationship between a patient and health professional and it is necessary to be attentive to health inequities.

Digital access to health, adjusting the oscillations between the decrease in cases, thanks to vaccination, and the occurrence of pandemic peaks in some places of the globe (such as China, January 2023), begins to be evidenced as one of the preferred means adopted by the population for their better access to health.

Naturally, the success rate and penetration will be higher in the younger, educated and lower digital illiteracy age groups.

The alternatives that are emerging in digital, through the advances of Augmented Reality and Virtual Reality Artificial Intelligence, contact devices such as chatbots and the focus on developing health applications that are easily navigable in mobile devices – *mobile-first sites and/*or APP's – will show strong growth in the coming years. By 2020, Portugal, with 11 million people, already had almost 16 million mobile phones, which translates into a great opening for an evolution in this direction.

Active Learning

Suggested Teaching Assignments.

If you attend higher education, try to know what projects are taking place at the institution or in your community considering digital health tools, research, and integrated interventions with health, social environment and education.

Share your findings with your research colleagues or other partners.

Web Search

Health literacy Portuguese scientific society: https://www.splsportugal.pt
Best apps for health and wellbeing: https://www.si.com/showcase/health/best-health-apps

Artificial Intelligence and Extended Reality: https://www.frontiersin.org/articles/10.3389/frvir.2021.721933/full

Exercise of Self-knowledge

Think about how many digital health solutions have appeared in recent times and make a list of innovative apps and describe advantages and barriers

References

Almeida, C. V. (2019). Modelo de comunicação em saúde ACP: As competências de comunicação no cerne de uma literacia em saúde transversal, holística e prática. In C. Lopes & C. V. Almeida (Coords.), *Literacia em saúde na prática* (pp. 43–52). Edições ISPA [ebook]. http://loja.ispa.pt/produto/literacia-em-saude-na-pratica

Almeida, C. V., Moraes, K. L., & Brasil, V. V. (2020). Introdução. In C. V. Almeida, K. L. Moraes & V. V. Brasil (Coords.), *50 Técnicas de literacia em saúde na prática. Um guia para a saúde* (pp. 8–12). Novas Edições Académicas.

Bandura, A. (Ed.). (1999). *Self-efficacy in changing societies*. Cambridge University Press.

Brach, C., Keller, D., Hernandez, L. M., Baur, C., Parker, R., Dreyer, B., Schyve, P., Lemerise, A. J., & Schillinger, D. (2012). Ten Attributes of Health Literate Health Care Organizations. NAM Perspectives. Discussion Paper, National Academy of Medicine, Washington, DC. https://doi.org/10.31478/201206a

Cacciamani, G. E., Shah, M., Yip, W., Abreu, A., Park, D., & Fuchs, G. (2020, July 27). Impact of Covid-19 on the urology service in United States: Perspectives and strategies to face a pandemic. *International Brazilien journal of Urology*, *46*(1), 207–214. https://doi.org/10.1590/s1677-5538.ibju.2020.s126

Change Healthcare. (2020). *The draw of frictionless healthcare 10 best practices for creating an outstanding digital patient experience*. [Online]. changehealthcare.com

Clement, J. (2019). *Facebook: Number of monthly active users worldwide 2008–2020*. https://www.statista.com/statistics/264810/number-of-monthly-active-facebook-users-worldwide/

Espanha, R., Ávila,P., & Mendes, R.V. (2016). Literacia em saúde em Portugal. Relatóro sintese. Lisboa. Fundação Calouste Gulbenkian.

European Commission. (2020a). *Three pillars to support our approach*. [Online]. https://ec.europa.eu/info/strategy/priorities-2019-2024/europe-fit-digital-age/shaping-europe-digital-future_en

European Commission. (2020b). *Shaping Europe's digital future: Commission presents strategies for data and Artificial Intelligence*. [Online]. https://ec.europa.eu/commission/presscorner/detail/en/ip_20_273

European Commission. (2020c). *Shaping Europe's digital future – Questions and answers*. [Online]. https://ec.europa.eu/digital-single-market/en/news/new-opportunities-digital-health-startups-and-smes

European Commission. (2020d). *New opportunities for digital health startups and SMEs*. [Online]. https://ec.europa.eu/commission/presscorner/detail/en/qanda_20_264

Ferreira, D. (2018). Teleconsultas: Ir ao hospital sem sair de casa implicações na relação médico-doente. *Medicina Interna*, *25*(1), 10–14. https://dx.doi.org/10.24950/rspmi/Opiniao/1/2018

Ferreira, F., Antunes, E., Neves, R. C., Farias, F., Malveiro, P., Choon, H., Galrinho, A., & Ferreira, R. C. (2012). Telemonitorização de INR: Eficácia e Segurança de um Sistema de Avaliação em 453 Doentes. *Acta Médica Portuguesa*, *25*(5), 297–300.

Influencer Marketing Hub. (2019). *75+ Social media sites you need to know in 2020*. https://influencermarketinghub.com/top-social-media-sites/

Jandoo, T. (2020). WHO guidance for digital health: What it means for researchers. *Digital Health, 6*, 2055207619898984. https://doi.org/10.1177/2055207619898984

Jiang, X., Deng, L, Zhu, Y., Ji, H., Tao, L., Liu, L., Yang, D., & Ji, W. (2020). Psychological crisis intervention during the outbreak period of new coronavirus pneumonia from experience in Shanghai. *Psychiatry Research, 286*, 112903. https://doi.org/10.1016/j.psychres.2020.112903

Kreps, G. L. (1988). Relational communication in health care. *Southern Speech Communication Journal, 53*, 344–359.

Lobban, F., Appelbe, D., Appleton, V., Aref-Adib, G., Barraclough, J., Billsborough, J., Fisher, N. R., Foster, S., Gill, B., Glentworth, D., Harrop, C., Johnson, S., Jones, S. H., Kovacs, T. Z., Lewis, E., Mezes, B., Morton, C., Murray, E., O'Hanlon, P., Pinfold, V., ... Wintermeyer, C. (2020). An online supported self-management toolkit for relatives of people with psychosis or bipolar experiences: The IMPART multiple case study. NIHR Journals Library. https://pubmed.ncbi.nlm.nih.gov/32986342/

Medeiros, L., Ferreira, H., & Júnior, G. (2020). Telemedicina – O "novo normal" do atendimento aos pacientes e colaboradores de centro oncohematológico, em tempos de Covid-19: Relato de experiência. *Hematology, Transfusion And Cell Therapy, 42*, 559. https://doi.org/10.1016/J.Htct.2020.10.944

Nissen, L., & Lindhardt, T. (2017). A qualitative study of COPD-patients' experience of a telemedicine intervention. *International Journal of Medical Informatics, 107*, 11–17. https://doi.org/10.1016/j.ijmedinf.2017.08.004

Pagoto, S., & Bennett, G. G. (2013). How behavioral science can advance digital health. *Translational Behavioral Medicine, 3*(3), 271–276. https://doi.org/10.1007/s13142-013-0234-z

Palmeira, C. S., Ramos, G. A., &, Mussi, F. C. (2020). Avaliação da experiência do telemonitoramento de enfermagem por mulheres com excesso de peso. *Escola Anna Nery, 25*(1), 1–8, e20200090. https://dx.doi.org/10.1590/2177-9465-ean-2020-0090

Ramos, S. (2020). Advocacia do paciente. In C. V. Almeida, K. L. Moraes, & V. V. Brasil (Coords.), *50 Técnicas de literacia em saúde na prática. Um guia para a saúde* (pp. 14–18). Novas Edições Académicas.

Reid Chassiakos, Y. L., Radesky, J., Christakis, D., Moreno, M. A., Cross, C., & Council on Communications and Media (2016). Children and Adolescents and Digital Media. *Pediatrics, 138*(5), e20162593. https://doi.org/10.1542/peds.2016-2593

Rodrigues, P. (2020). Repetição. In C. V. Almeida, K. Moraes, & V. V. Brasil (Coords.), *50 Técnicas de literacia em saúde na prática. Um guia para a saúde* (pp. 93–94). Novas Edições Académicas.

Serafini, G., Parmigiani, B., Amerio, A., Aguglia, A., Sher, L., & Amore, M. (2020). The psychological impact of COVID-19 on the mental health in the general population. *QJM: An International Journal of Medicine*. https://doi.org/10.1093/qjmed/hcaa201

SNS 24. (2019). *A solidão e o isolamento social*. https://www.sns24.gov.pt/guia/a-solidao-e-o-isolamento-social/

Sørensen, K., Van den Broucke, S., Fullam, J., Doyle, G., Pelikan, J., Slonska, Z., Brand, H., & (HLS-EU) Consortium Health Literacy Project European, (2012). Health literacy and public health: a systematic review and integration of definitions and models. *BMC public health, 12*, 80. https://doi.org/10.1186/1471-2458-12-80

Tench, R., & Konczos, M. (2013). *Mapping European communication practitioners' competencies: A review of the European communication professional skills and innovation program*. ECOPSI.

Thakur, B., & Pathak, M. (2021). Burden of predominant psychological reactions among the healthcare workers and general during COVID-19 pandemic phase: A systematic review and meta-analysis. Project: Mental Health during COVID-19 Pandemic phase (License CC BY 4.0). https://doi.org/10.1101/2021.01.02.21249126

Van Lieshout, F., Yang, R., Stamenova, V., Agarwal, P., Cornejo Palma, D., Sidhu, A., Engel, K., Erwood, A., Bhatia, R. S., Bhattacharyya, O., & Shaw J. (2020). Evaluating the implementation of a remote-monitoring program for chronic obstructive pulmonary disease: Qualitative methods from a service design perspective. *Journal of Medical Internet Research, 22*(10), e18148. https://doi.org/10.2196/18148

Viana, R. B., & Lira, C. A. B. (2020). Exergames as coping strategies for anxiety disorders during the COVID-19 quarantine period. *Games Health Journal, 9*(3), 1–3. https://doi.org/10.1089/g4h.2020.0060

Vaz de Almeida, C. (2020a). *Organizações e profissionais de saúde: E depois, continuamos no digital? A Pátria.* https://apatria.org/autor/vazdealmeidacristinagmail-com/

Vaz de Almeida, C. (2020b). Organizações literadas, literacia em saúde e boas práticas em tempo de pandemia – ao encontro dos objetivos do desenvolvimento sustentável. *APDH* [Online]. https://www.apdh.pt/artigo/67

Waller, G., Pugh, M., Mulkens, S., Moore, E., Mountford, V. A., Carter, J., Wicksteed, A., Maharaj, A., Wade, T. D., Wisniewski, L., Farrell, N. R., Raykos, B., Jorgensen, S., Evans, J., Thomas, J. J., Osenk, I., Paddock, C., Bohrer, B., Anderson, K., Turner, H., … Smit, V. (2020). Cognitive-behavioral therapy in the time of coronavirus: Clinician tips for working with eating disorders via telehealth when face-to-face meetings are not possible. *International Journal Eating Disorder*, 1–10. https://doi.org/10.1002/eat.23289

WHO. (2023). *World Health Organization Coronavirus disease (COVID-19) Dashboard.* https://covid19.who.int/ Acedido em 4 fevereiro 2023

WHO. (2020). *Quality Assurance, Norms and Standards.* https://www.who.int/our-work/science-division/quality-assurance-norms-and-standards

WONCA. (2002). *Definição europeia de medicina geral e familiar (Clínica Geral/Medicina Familiar).* WONCA.

Zhang, J., Wu, W., Zhao, X., & Zhang, W. (2020). Recommended psychological crisis intervention response to the 2019 novel coronavirus pneumonia outbreak in China: A model of West China Hospital. *Precision Clinical Medicine, 3*(1), 3–8. https://doi.org/10.1093/pcmedi/pbaa006

Chapter 2

Forty Definitions and Metaphors for Active and Transormative Learning in Chat GPT Times: Chat GPT as an Active and Transformative Technology Enhanced Learning Boost in Healthcare Education

Miltiadis D. Lytras[a,b]

[a]*Effat Univerity, Effat College of Engineering, Effat, Saudi Arabia*
[b]*MIS Department, The American College of Greece, Athens, Greece*

Abstract

Healthcare education is a huge industry with a significant social footprint and resilient impact on well-being and on the quality of life. It integrates diverse scientific domains and needs to continuously update its value proposition to reflect the need for preparing top-quality health professionals. It also has to support professional development and to manage effectively the accreditation of programs and the certification of skills and knowledge. In this chapter, the authors expand a theoretical framework about Active and Transformative Learning (ATL) that has introduced in the volume of ATL for STEAM disciplines and also discussed how artificial intelligent (AI) tools, such as OPENAI Chat GPT, can serve as transformers and value carriers for the implementation of ATL activities and use cases in healthcare education.

Keywords: Active learning; transformative learning; healthcare education; Next Generation HealthCare; artificial intelligence; Chat GPT; OpenAI

Technology-Enhanced Healthcare Education:
Transformative Learning for Patient-Centric Health, 19–34
Copyright © 2024 by Miltiadis D. Lytras
Published under exclusive licence by Emerald Publishing Limited
doi:10.1108/978-1-83753-598-920231002

1. Introduction – A 5-Tier ATL Framework for Exploitation in Healthcare Education

The use of learning technologies in education is an old story. During the last 50 years, new technologies always supported efficiently educational strategies and also serves learners with tools, services and innovative pedagogical approaches. In the last couple years, a lot of discussion is made about the disruptive and transformative character of AI and tools like OpenAI Chat GPT.

In an effort to communicate in this chapter some thoughts about the capacity of Chat GPT technology to serve the ATL strategy, we will build on a 5-tier framework introduced in a complementary edition by Lytras (2023).

In the basic abstraction of the framework, five strategic pillars provide the value components of an ATL Framework, namely:

- Active and Transformative Learning
- Higher education
- Entrepreneurship
- Industry
- Research and innovation

Additionally, for the ATL pillar, eight additional value carriers and areas of special interests were identified including:

- Knowledge and content
- Learning strategies
- Technology enhanced learning enhancement
- Skills and competencies uniqueness
- Faculty capacity to implement
- Administrative support and educational leadership
- Impact measurement and learning analytics

The healthcare education industry can exploit these theoretical abstractions towards the design and implementation of a Technology Enhanced Active and Transformative Learning (TEATL) Strategy. The overall idea is that a resilient TEATL STRATEGY IN Healthcare Education has to integrate the interests and the objectives of five types of diverse stakeholders, namely: ATL, Higher Education (HE), Entrepreneurship, Industry, and Research and Innovation.

The effort to provide a systematic ontological discussion on the ATL is not a simple task. The complexity of the Learning domain, the diverse theories and the background disciplines make this intellectual task even more difficult. In our approach, we investigate how some of the following research and scientific domains interact in order to support a new value proposition for ATL in education:

- Learning Designs (Naeve et al., 2008).
- Knowledge and Learning Management (Lytras et al., 2005).

- Social Media (Lytras & de Pablos, 2009; Lytras et al., 2018c; Zhuhadar et al., 2013).
- Data Science and Analytics (Arafat et al., 2019).
- Sustainable Management of Higher Education in times of crisis and multifold challenges (Al-Youbi et al., 2020).
- Emerging Technologies, for example, AI, Metaverse, Virtual Reality, Cloud computing (Lytras et al., 2018a, 2018b; Zhang et al., 2017b).
- Transformative Leadership in Education.
- Educational strategies at national and institutional levels (Lytras & Mathkour, 2017; Lytras et al., 2016; Zhang et al., 2017).
- Smart Education and Digital Transformation (Lytras & Visvizi, 2020; Lytras et al., 2019; Visvizi & Lytras, 2018).

In this chapter, we try to communicate one more piece of wisdom for our foundations on ATL. In Section 2, we elaborate the ontological definitions and metaphors of the ATL introduced by Lytras (2023), while in Section 3 we communicate how Chat GPT can serve such a framework with tools and services to be integrated into Healthcare Education.

2. Forty Definitions and Metaphors for Active Learning

ATL, according to Lytras (2023b), is a multidimensional value space with multiple reference theories and background disciplines. In this section, we provide an ontological approach to the phenomenon aiming to discuss some of its facets, for further exploitation. Lytras (2023) proposed 23 metaphors of the phenomenon, and in this section we expand and summarize 12 more. In fact, we define a 40-axis value space for the implementation of Active and Transformative Learning in Education. Each dimension and value-axis can also be exploited for the parameterization of the ATL strategy.

2.1 Definitions and Metaphors of ATL With Emphasis on Learning Dimension

Our proposition on ATL is based on an ontological framework that has been defined in Lytras (2023). In fact, our approach provides a contextual framework for the identification of the core elements of the unique value proposition of the ATL strategy. In this section, we elaborate the seven core components related to the learning and educational dimension of our ALT theory.

Pillar 1. Knowledge and Content

Definition 1. ATL as a holistic paradigm for learning content and knowledge packaging:

ATL among other priorities is also focusing on the sophisticated learning content and knowledge packaging in ways and modes that promoted and enhance the learning impact and the value of the learning experiences. It is related to the extensive use of templates, metadata and content unit structures that have the capacity to offer dynamic modes of content exploration.

Definition 2. ATL as a dynamic, fully personalized knowledge exploration strategy for multidimensional learning impact:

The ATL paradigm allows multiple modes of knowledge and context exploration and utilization, with an enhanced multidimensional learning impact. For this purpose deploys infrastructures, services and context exploitation templates that allow personalized learning paths, sophisticated learning content retrieval, dynamic composition of education and training modules, and on-demand learning experiences.

Definition 3. ATL as a data-driven knowledge and learning dissemination paradigm:

ATL on its full utilization and scope has a robust data ecosystem of learning resources, knowledge and learning dissemination mechanisms and services. It consists of a sophisticated ecosystem of value-adding learning services that are data-driven and attached to learning content that has been carefully prepared and packaged to adopt the ATL strategy.

Definition 4. ATL as a robust modular learning content learning development path:

The ATL is a fully integrative developmental path for individuals and teams that is supported by robust modular learning content utilization. In fact, the ATL is exploiting microcontents, templates and standardized databases of structured and unstructured learning content that can be multipurposely integrated into meaningful learning paths.

Pillar 2. Learning Strategies

Definition 5. ATL as a unified learning strategy for multidimensional learning impact:

ATL is overall a unified learning strategy for the realization of multidimensional learning impact. It integrates components that target a holistic impact by building connectors and multipliers between different stakeholders from the HE, the industry, the entrepreneurship, the innovation, the research and development (R&D) and the social areas.

Definition 6. ATL as an innovative and integrated knowledge utilization context for HE, industry, entrepreneurship, innovation, R&D and social impact:

ATL is putting together a shared vision and responsibility of HE among six different types of stakeholders and communities of shared interests. ATL is an innovative and integrated knowledge utilization context for HE, industry, entrepreneurship, innovation, R&D and social impact. In other words, the learning context of the ATL cultivates and strengthens the impact of the learning experience by building greater association and relevance to the interest of diverse communities and external stakeholders.

Definition 7. ATL as a new proposition for a holistic taxonomy of (learning) objectives:

In our theoretical abstraction, ATL is a new proposition for a holistic taxonomy of value objectives including learning objectives as well as objectives related to the industry alignment, promotion of entrepreneurship, enhancement of innovation, support of R&D, and social impact.

Pillar 3. Technology Enhanced Learning Enhancement

Definition 8. ATL as a unique test-bed for the exploitation of emerging technologies such as AI, Metaverse, Cloud computing, Educational Portfolios, Open educational resources, Learning Objects, etc.:

ATL is also innovating in the way that is exploiting and deploying diverse learning technologies in order to enrich the learning experience and to get value of their synthesis. ATL is a holistic strategy for managing the portfolio of Technology Enhanced Tools and Services with a clear strategic orientation.

Definition 9. ATL as an overarching principle of Technology-enhanced active learning initiatives:

ATL unifies the technology enhanced active learning initiatives and strategizes the value propositions of each component to the overall strategic targets and objectives. Thus, the technology enablement is justified and reasoned on the basis of a concrete pedagogical philosophy and paradigm.

Pillar 4. Skills and Competencies Uniqueness

Definition 10. ATL as a sustainable mechanism for skills and competencies elevation:

ATL is focusing on the elevation of skills and competencies. Has a strong orientation to the development of all aspects of personality and a complete set of complementary skills and competencies. For this purpose, the full ATL ecosystem is maintaining and exploiting a sustainable data warehouse of skills and competencies.

Definition 11. ATL as a plain strategy for building a resilient competence to learn:

One of the greatest features and gains of ATL is its capacity to support individual, teams and organizations to develop a competence to learn and to adopt. This is a systemic added value of the ATL strategy, and is supported by all the other value components of our ATL theory.

Pillar 5. Faculty Capacity to Implement

Definition 12. ATL as a resilient faculty empowerment ecosystem:

The ATL is a resilient and progressive faculty empowerment ecosystem. It uses methods and procedures for faculty profiling, assessment, readiness, development and quality.

Definition 13. ATL as a bold approach for exploiting the faculty's learning creativity and responsibility:

ATL is providing a full strategy for exploiting the faculty learning creativity by promoting co-design and co-responsibility in the crafting and the implementation of the strategy. It also rewards faculty for the commitment, unique achievement and contributions to the overall ATL milestones.

Pillar 6. Administrative Support and Educational Leadership

Definition 14. ATL as a sustainable and evolutionary Education Leadership paradigm:

The ATL strategy has a bold component of Administrative Support and Educational Leadership. It comes with bold proposition for the new leadership required by academic administrators and educational administrators in order to support the overall philosophy and strategy. It is based on co-design and co-responsibility.

Pillar 7. Impact Measurement & Learning Analytics

Definition 15. ATL as an integrated Impact and Learning Analytics multi-instrument in higher education:

ATL is utilizing an integrated Impact and Learning Analytics multi-instrument in HE. Within the ATL ecosystem special emphasis is paid to the definition, maintenance and measurement of metrics, key performance indicators, benchmarks and analytics related to diverse and complimentary facets of the ATL strategy. This ontological feature of the ATL directly connects the strategy with an operational, daily process of recording, and measuring data elements attach to the value ecosystem of ATL.

Definition 16. ATL as an institutional wide spectrum of milestones and achievements:

ATL is oriented to a full set of milestones related to the actualization of its added value and the realization of its full potential and impact.

Definition 17. ATL as a progressive evolutionary maturity achievement framework:

ATL is a holistic strategy, that is, visioning different maturity levels related to its implementation and impact. It offers to institutions a scalable approach of impact, excellence and achievements.

In Fig. 2.1, we summarize the 17 definitions and metaphors of the ATL with a focus on the learning dimension and the learning impact.

2.2. Definitions and Metaphors of ATL With Emphasis on Higher Education, Industry, and R&D and Innovation

In the previous section, we provided some ontological classification for the philosophy and the paradigm of the ATL. In this section, we expand further our

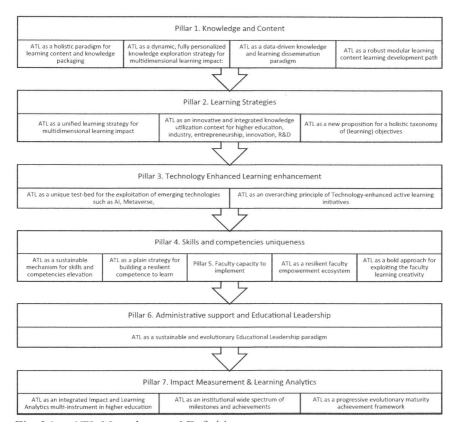

Fig. 2.1.   ATL Metaphors and Definitions.

theoretical abstraction for ATL emphasizing on the other four components of our methodological framework, namely: Higher Education, Industry, Entrepreneurship, and R&D and Innovation.

1. *ATL as a bold strategy and differentiation factor in HE institutions*

The ATL is related to a bold strategy that can be used for the re-positioning of the value proposition of all the educational institutions. ATL strategy includes vision, mission and action plans that jointly formulate the strategic house and the strategic objectives of the entire strategy.

2. *ATL as a core positioning and differentiating factor in the HE industry/Market*

ATL is a complex set of interconnecting processes, and value activities, a unique educational mix that can be customized for a strategic positioning in the Higher Education and Education industry and Market. Towards this direction institutions and administrators have to identify, support and communicate the robust ATL educational mix and strategy to all the stakeholders.

3. *ATL as a core pillar of Faculty Development Programs*

ATL is a critical pillar of Faculty Development programs, providing a holistic approach for the development of skills and competencies of faculty for the design and adoption in the daily educational and learning practice of resilient activities. From this perspective, ATL is an overarching principle for the direction and the objectives of the faculty development programs especially those targeting a 360 degrees approach to the development.

4. *ATL strategy as a vital enabler or 360 degrees enrichment of value proposition in HE*

ATL is a holistic and vital enabler of 360 degrees enrichment of the value proposition in HE including a complete set of Key performance Indicators, analytics and value core components that justify a robust educational and learning value chain.

5. *ATL as a unique learning setting for talent identification, development and exploitation*

ATL has a unique orientation to talent identification, development and exploitation. It serves as a sustainable, resilient and robust integrated approach for a learning-based exploratory talent management. It has the capacity to promote the individual, team and institutional talent.

6. *ATL as a holistic strategy for skills and competencies development*

ATL is an end-to-end, institutional-wide holistic strategy for skills and competencies identification, assessment, elevation and development with clear linkage to the industry and market needs. It utilizes an integrated standardization of skills and competencies elements and constructively promotes their elevation.

7. *ATL as a reward and incentive mechanism for faculty to promote ALT in learning delivery*

ATL is promoting a holistic rewards and incentives mechanism for faculty as champions of ATL in real educational settings. From this perspective, ATL integrates well-defined supporting and reward procedures to the faculty and sets milestones and benchmarks for achievements.

8. *ATL as a holistic approach for the development of new skills and competencies*

ATL is a unique pedagogical and educational approach for the transformation of methods and tools for acquiring new skills and competencies. It is about deploying tools and services for skills and competencies out of the box. It is a primer of education out-of-the-box.

9. *ATL as a bold approach/paradigm shift for a new generation of learning matched to the industry needs*

ATL is a unique paradigm shift for a new generation of learning experiences and learning paths tailored made to match the needs of learners, groups and institutions imposed by the industry needs. ATL offers a synchronization of real-world needs with the content and the process of learning and education.

10. *ATL as an integral and interconnected ecosystem of resources for dynamic learning spaces, technology enhanced and tailored to the needs of individuals and teams*

ATL provides an integral and interconnected ecosystem of resources for dynamic learning spaces, technology enhanced and tailored to the needs of individuals and teams. In other words, the ATL provides the dynamic and customizable backbone of learning content, processes and spaces that is technologically enhanced and meets the needs of all the stakeholders. The development of the ATL infrastructure both from procedural and technological point of view are integral parts of an effective ATL strategy.

11. *ATL as a primer of robust expertise transfer*

ATL has a unique capacity and an integral procedural system that promotes robust expertise transfer. The emphasis of ATL on the know-how transfer is bringing together academia, industry and innovation, and utilizes novel pedagogical methods and techniques.

12. *ATL as an innovative technique for future jobs training*

ATL has a unique capacity to adopt its methodologies for future job training. By introducing innovative learning methods and educational labs, and by designing use cases for the use of emerging multi- and interdisciplinary training, ATL has the capacity to support effectively educational curricula related to future jobs.

13. *ATL as a transformative educational and learning paradigm for a new era of value proposition in HE*

ATL is not a repetition or integration of existing learning approaches. Is a brand new transformative educational, learning paradigm that challenges traditional and established learning and educational strategies, methodologies, and practices. It introduces a new era of learner-centric development with value delivery anchored in five areas (education, industry, innovation, entrepreneurship, and R&D capability).

14. *ATL as an approach for continuous personal and professional development*

ATL offers a powerful and resilient methodology for continuous personal and professional development. It is equipped with diverse and complementary activities, processes and methods that allow individuals and professionals to build sustainable development learning programs and paths. At an institutional level ATL also offers a new channel for delivery of educational programs and modules.

15. *ATL as a holistic strategy for development of critical thinking capability of students*

ATL promotes a wide range of educational and learning objectives but focuses on the development of the critical thinking capability of students. For this purpose, it utilizes technology enhanced learning, creative ideas on instructional design and dynamic, and flexible learning experiences.

16. *ATL as a multidimensional/360 degrees approach for identification and management of talent of young people*

ATL is aiming to support young talented students that are struggled by monolithic educational activities and rigid educational curricula. From this point of view, it offers a multidimensional/360 degrees approach for the identification and management of talent of young people.

17. *ATL as a unique value proposition for the integration as Generalized Pretrained Transformers from AI domain*

ATL is a unified test-bed for the exploitation of transformative pretrained transformers, for example, OpenAI CHAT GPT, in the domain of technology-enhanced learning. ATL exploits different GPT services and use cases for the realization of value for learners and teams of learners as well as faculty. In the next section of this chapter, we provide few ideas on how Chat GPT can serve as a role model for ATL assignments.

18. *ATL as a strategy to promote start-ups student-driven ecosystem*

ATL is cultivating a culture and formulating a strategy to promote and strengthen the student-driven start-ups ecosystem. In other words, ATL serves as a bold enabler of creative ideas of students for innovation, entrepreneurship and start-ups. In such a context, HE has to define procedures, assessments and programs that target on intellectual milestones, such as start-ups and business plans for innovations.

19. *ATL as a catalyst for technology transfer of research and knowledge-based innovation*

ATL is a catalyst for the technology transfer of research and knowledge-based innovation. The overall idea is that the overarching ATL strategy mobilizes resources and provides channels that allow a resilient technology transfer of research outputs, innovations, and R&D artefacts and services. In the current version of the educational systems, it is really hard to see this process prioritized and implemented as a bold aspect of the unique value proposition of the institutions.

20. *ATL as a multiplier of intrinsic motivation for research and development for individuals, teams and institutions*

ATL has unique features, exploratory methods and engaging contexts that promote and enhance the intrinsic motivation for R&D of individuals and teams. ATL is about enhancing the capacity of people to learn and to deliver high-quality research. It is a critical paradigm shift on the underlying philosophy of learning to learn more effectively.

21. *ATL as a key pillar of the research infrastructure in colleges and universities*

ATL can be seen as an absolute and substantial pillar of the research infrastructure in colleges and universities. By providing unique methods and services for research capacity building and by putting together individuals' skills and competencies in greater contexts of exploitation, ATL initiates a new era of flexible research infrastructures in colleges and universities.

22. *ATL as a core component of the R&D and Innovation Strategy in HE institutions*

ATL is not an isolated strategy. An alternative way to consider its unique value proposition is by considering it as a core component of the R&D and Innovation Strategy in HE institutions. ATL must serve the R&D Process and Function in HE institutions and in parallel should also provide an end-to-end mode of enormous, excessive R&D capability on demand. ATL is thus offering a dynamic context for exploiting individual research skills and competence, and transforming them to institutional research excellence.

23. *ATL as a vehicle for the resilient transferring of research skills, research methodologies, etc.*

ATL is a transparent vehicle for the resilient transferring of research skills, research methodologies and research competence. In this direction, ATL is exploiting numerous methodological approaches for knowledge transfer, research capacity building and research empowerment. In the context of HE institutions, this principle should be transparent and diffused across all academic programs and curricula.

3. Chat GPT as an Enabler ATL Metaphors

The Chat GPT represents a new generation of technologies that challenge not only education but the entire well-established way of human–computer interaction. It is about a brand new way of knowledge filtering, structuring and use. In this section, we provide some ideas on how a disruptive technology like Chat GPR can also serve the purposes and the strategic orientation of ATL in HE and in healthcare education. We selected few scenarios in Table 2.1, while in a future publication, we will provide a more integrated and complete overview.

Table 2.1.   ChatGPT as an Enabler for ATL.

ATL Metaphor Definition	Chat GPT Utilization Scenario/Use Case
Pillar 1. Knowledge and Content	
ATL as a holistic paradigm for learning content and knowledge packaging	• Chat GPT as a tool to package learning modules, and learning objects from open educational repositories • Chat GPT as a polymorphic tool for knowledge discovery and composition • Chat GPT as a unique tool for preparing assignments and assessments with an emphasis on Bloom's Taxonomy of Learning Objectives

(Continued)

Table 2.1.   (*Continued*)

ATL Metaphor Definition	Chat GPT Utilization Scenario/Use Case
ATL as a dynamic, fully personalized knowledge exploration strategy for multidimensional learning impact	• Chat GTP as a unified model for designing learning paths and supportive content modules • Chat GPT as a tool for matching skills and competencies with knowledge items and assignments • Chat GPT as a holistic measurable exploratory context for team collaboration in universities
ATL as a data-driven knowledge and learning dissemination paradigm	• Chat GPT as a robust knowledge drill-down tool • Chat GPT as a data miner of meaningful knowledge and learning modules • Chat GPT as a pre-human pre-processing level for learning content authoring
ATL as a robust modular learning content learning development path	• Chat GPT as a scalable exploratory mechanism for the body of knowledge in any domain • Chat GPT as a customizable knowledge abstraction and extendable development path
Pillar 2. Learning Strategies	
ATL as a unified learning strategy for multidimensional learning impact	• Chat GPT as a tool to analyze the core value components of multidimensional learning impact with emphasis on an ontological agreement
ATL as an innovative and integrated knowledge utilization context for higher education, industry, entrepreneurship, innovation, R&D and social impact	• Chat GPT as a resilient platform for new knowledge generation for bridging education, industry and innovation curricula • Chat GPT as a distiller of interdisciplinary and multidisciplinary curricula
ATL as a new proposition for a holistic taxonomy of (learning) objectives	• Chat GPT as a model platform for promoting learning objectives using the 40-tier approach discussed in our methodological framework • Chat GPT as a learning tool to prepare modules for diverse and scalable learning objectives • Chat GPT as a miner of matching the needs of industry, R&D and innovation, and the unique value propositions of educational curricula

Table 2.1. (*Continued*)

ATL Metaphor Definition	Chat GPT Utilization Scenario/Use Case
Pillar 3. Technology Enhanced Learning Enhancement	
ATL as a unique test-bed for the exploitation of emerging technologies such as AI, Metaverse, etc.	• Chat GPT as a test bed for the use of AI in all the aspects of educational programs design, implementation and evaluation • Chat GPR as a scripting power-house for learning content
ATL as an overarching principle of technology-enhanced active learning initiatives	• Chat GPT as a dynamic instrument for designing learning stories, use cases, learning scenarios and learning contexts

4. Discussion and Conclusions

The ontological discussion of the ATL in the previous section serves three critical objectives:

• To introduce a methodological framework with clear reference to the various value core components of the ATL.
• To provide an ontological agreement on the key aspects of the phenomenon, by introducing, complementary facets.
• To provide an extendable working set of principles and basic assumptions for our unique value proposition on the ATL.

It is obvious that the exhaustive discussion of our theoretical proposition needs further elaboration. The 40 metaphors and definitions introduced in this section as parts of an integrated ATL strategy need further detailing and hermeneutic and operational/functional instruments and tools. We intend in our next planned editions to provide additional details about this approach and also to communicate evidence from the adoption of our key principles in real educational settings.

As a concluding remark of this chapter, we had to emphasize that ATL is a holistic paradigm, with a solid theoretical multidisciplinary background and with a robust strategy that implements procedures, action plans, learning impact and unique learning experiences. It offers a unique amalgam for the synchronization and the utilization of higher education, industry, innovation, entrepreneurship, R&D capability and social impact.

REFERENCES

AI-Youbi, A. O., Al-Hayani, A., Bardesi, H. J., Basheri, M., Lytras, M. D., & Aljohani, N. R. (2020). The King Abdulaziz University (KAU) pandemic framework: A methodological approach to leverage social media for the sustainable management of higher education in crisis. Sustainability, 12(11), 4367.

Arafat, S., Aljohani, N., Abbasi, R., Hussain, A., & Lytras, M. (2019). Connections between e-learning, web science, cognitive computation and social sensing, and their relevance to learning analytics: A preliminary study. *Computers in Human Behavior*, *92*, 478–486.

Lytras, M. (2023). Active and Transformative Learning (ATL) in Higher Education in times of Artificial Intelligence and ChatGPT: Investigating a value-based framework. In Lytras (Ed.), *Active and transformative learning in STEAM disciplines: From curriculum design to social impact*, (pp. 5-24). Emerald Publishing Limited, ISBN: 9781837536191.

Lytras, M., & Housawi, A. (2023). Active Learning in Healthcare Education, Training and Research: A Digital Transformation primer. In Lytras & Vaz De Almeida (Eds.), Active Learning for Digital Transformation in Healthcare Education, Training and Research (Next Generation Technology Driven Personalized Medicine and Smart Healthcare). Elsevier: Academic Press. ISBN: 9780443152481

Lytras, M. D., Aljohani, N. R., Visvizi, A., Ordonez De Pablos, P., & Gasevic, D. (2018a). Advanced decision-making in higher education: Learning analytics research and key performance indicators.*Behaviour & Information Technology*, *37*(10–11), 937–940. https://doi.org/10.1080/0144929X.2018.1512940

Lytras, M. D., Damiani, E., & Mathkour, H. (2016). Virtual reality in learning, collaboration and behaviour: Content, systems, strategies, context designs. *Behaviour and Information Technology*, *35*(11), 877–878. https://doi.org/10.1080/0144929X.2016.1235815

Lytras, M. D., & de Pablos, P. O. (2009). *Social web evolution: Integrating semantic applications*. IGI Global. https://doi.org/10.4018/978-1-60566-272-5

Lytras, M. D., & Mathkour, H. (2017). Advances in research in social networking for open and distributed learning. *International Review of Research in Open and Distance Learning*, *18*(1), i–iv.

Lytras, M. D., Naeve, A., & Pouloudi, A. (2005). A knowledge management roadmap for e-learning: The way ahead. *International Journal of Distance Education Technologies*, *3*(2),68–75.

Lytras, M. D., & Visvizi, A. (2020). Big data research for social science and social impact. *Sustainability*, *12*, 180.

Lytras, M. D., Visvizi, A., Damiani, D., & Mthkour, H. (2018b). The cognitive computing turn in education: prospects and application.*Computers in Human Behavior*. https://doi.org/10.1016/j.chb.2018.11.011

Lytras, M. D., Visvizi, A., Daniela, L., Sarirete, A., & Ordonez De Pablos, P. (2018c). Social networks research for sustainable Smart education.*Sustainability*, *10*(9), 2974. https://doi.org/10.3390/su10092974

Lytras, M. D., Visvizi, A., & Sarirete, A. (2019). Clustering Smart City Services: Perceptions, expectations, responses.Sustainability, 11(6), 1669. https://doi.org/10.3390/su11061669

Naeve, A., Sicilia, M.-A., & Lytras, M. D. (2008). Learning processes and processing learning: From organizational needs to learning designs. *Journal of Knowledge Management*, *12*(6), 5–14. https://doi.org/10.1108/13673270810913586

Visvizi, A., & Lytras, M. D. (2018). Editorial: Policy making for Smart Cities: Innovation and social inclusive economic growth for sustainability.*Journal of Science and Technology Policy Management*, *9*, 126–133.

Zhang, X., Jiang, S., Ordonez de Pablos, P., Lytras, M. D., & Sun, Y. (2017). How virtual reality affects perceived learning effectiveness: A task's technology fit perspective. *Behaviour and Information Technology*, *36*(5), 548–556. https://doi.org/10.1080/0144929X.2016.1268647

Zhang, X., Zhang, Y., Sun, Y., Lytras, M., Ordonez de Pablos, P., & He, W. (2017b). Exploring the effect of transformational leadership on individual creativity in e-learning: a perspective of social exchange theory. *Studies in Higher Education*, 1–15. (in press). https://doi.org/10.1080/03075079.2017.1296824

Zhuhadar, L., Yang, R., & Lytras, M. D. (2013). The impact of social multimedia systems on cyberlearners. *Computers in Human Behavior*, *29*(2), 378–385.

Appendix: Case Study 1

Jenny is a Higher Education Consultant, responsible for crafting a strategy in a University for the integration of Chat GPT in the learning process. According to the Lytras (2023) framework, four more pillars are the value carriers for the ATL strategy:

Pillar 4. Skills and Competencies Uniqueness

- ATL as a sustainable mechanism for skills and competencies elevation
- ATL as a plain strategy for building a resilient competence to learn

Pillar 5. Faculty Capacity to Implement

- ATL as a resilient faculty empowerment ecosystem
- ATL as a bold approach for exploiting the faculty learning creativity and responsibility

Pillar 6. Administrative Support and Educational Leadership

- ATL as a sustainable and evolutionary Educational Leadership paradigm

Pillar 7. Impact Measurement & Learning Analytics

- ATL as an integrated Impact and Learning Analytics multi-instrument in higher education
- ATL as an institutional wide spectrum of milestones and achievements
- ATL as a progressive evolutionary maturity achievement framework

Questions

1. Can you propose one scenario for the utilization of the Chat GPT for these pillars?
2. Can you use Chat GPT and provide some evidence or use case for the implementation of your idea?
3. Which are the risks for using Chat GPT for the implementation of the ATL strategies and metaphors?
4. Can you draft on your own a scenario in one page for a template for a learning module that will integrate the ATL parading? Ask the same from Chat GPT and compare the two developments.

Topics for Essays or Assignments

1. ATL as a business model for a new era of educational services in Higher Education
2. ATL as a separate function in Centers of Teaching and Learning Excellence in universities and colleges
3. Chat GPT as a threat and as an opportunity for value-based education

Chapter 3

Mental Health and Higher Education Institutions: Next Steps to Well-being

Isabel Maria Abreu Rodrigues Fragoeiro

University of Madeira – Escola Superior de Saúde, Funchal, Portugal

Abstract

Learning to be someone in today's world requires training, knowledge, adaptive skills, differentiated skills, and mastery of instrumental and advanced technological tools to manage complex, new, and crucial problems that societies face. Citizens need to satisfy their basic needs, and they want to feel fulfilled. These are determinants of mental health/health, essential goods for the growth and evolution of humanity, and for the survival of the planet that shelters it.

The objectives of this chapter are: (1) reflect on the influence of mental health/health in high-level training processes, which require the student to mobilize physical and mental capabilities and functions; (2) realize to what extent the use of digital technology is an essential tool for learning and developing skills for higher education students; (3) addressing the question: Are higher education institutions (HEIs) and professors prepared for the challenges they face today? And, at the confluence of the previous three: (4) analyze the health/mental health interconnections, the use of digital technologies and training paths, as pillars of human development and the progress of societies.

In HEIs, there is evidence of the intersection of students' learning abilities with the contexts that are favourable to them, namely, due to the possibility of finding space to create, develop potentials, acquire high-level knowledge and skills, present themselves to society as reliable, credible, and promising professionals for success in the organizations they form part of.

For the preparation of this exploratory and reflective chapter, the collaboration of some higher education teachers in the Autonomous Region of Madeira

Technology-Enhanced Healthcare Education:
Transformative Learning for Patient-Centric Health, 35–46
Copyright © 2024 by Isabel Maria Abreu Rodrigues Fragoeiro
Published under exclusive licence by Emerald Publishing Limited
doi:10.1108/978-1-83753-598-920231003

(RAM) was requested, also basing it on their own experience and knowledge acquired as a teacher, researcher, and expert in the field of mental health.

The perspective presented for reflection and analysis is limited by the look and the way we interrogate and interpret the realities where we operate, for these same reasons, imbued with subjectivity.

Keywords: Mental health; higher education; digital technologies; interconnections; integral development; health education

Mental Health and Higher Education

In recent years, mental health and the various teaching contexts have been recurrently interconnected, especially in HEIs, which was greatly accentuated with the pandemic by SARS CoV 2. In developed societies, the incidence and prevalence of psycho-emotional and mental disorders have increased (WHO, 2022), including young people and young adults, showing that their implications in teaching–learning processes have been the subject of attention and studies in several regions and countries, including Europe (Carette et al., 2018; JISC, 2020; Royal College of Psychiatrists, 2011, 2020; Tabor et al., 2021; Zapata-Garibay et al., 2021). In Portugal, several initiatives related to the study/assessment of lifestyles, well-being, and mental health of higher education students have been carried out, and HEIs located in several different regions of the country, projects that promote well-being and mental health, including the RAM (Academic Association of the University of Madeira, 2022; Comprehensive Health Research Centre, 2022; Coordinating Council of Polytechnic Higher Institutes (CCISP), 2021; Council Rectors of Portuguese Universities, 2021; Sequeira et al., 2020; Sequeira & Sampaio, 2020; University of Madeira, Psychology Service, 2022).

In fact, psychological suffering and frustration caused by insecurity and lack of freedom unprecedented in the last century have increased significantly, leaving individuals more vulnerable to the development of mental health problems (Zapata-Garibay et al., 2021).

This trend was particularly felt in the academic community, where the COVID-19 pandemic has generated uncertainty and increased stress. It should also be noted that three quarters of all mental changes throughout life occur before the age of 25, and adolescents and young people are increasingly likely to report mental health problems (Tabor et al., 2021).

Different members of the academies are currently more sensitive to the need for and importance of, in these contexts, implementing interventions aimed at creating environments that promote health, mental health, and collective well-being.

We are also at a stage in the evolutionary paths of academic contexts and social contexts (referring to the more developed countries), in which unsatisfied needs are identified, regarding the mental health of students and other members of HEIs, which is considered of great importance for a more focused and in-depth reflection on what can be done and how we can act in order to obtain health gains. Not only with the participation of members of academia, but also with those professionals who, being holders of differentiated knowledge and skills in mental health and with a perspective of community mental health, can contribute to an appropriate intervention to minimize difficulties and problems that are identified and diagnosed, and can be addressed or even resolved.

Access to higher education continues to represent a desired expectation for many young people and young adults. It is also known that, in a lifelong development process, in which the need to adapt to rapid social and work changes is increasingly evident, the number of adults of various ages who attend higher education has increased. Senior universities are also illustrative of this demand for updating and training, both individually and collectively, at more advanced ages.

Nowadays, along with the satisfaction of personal expectations, the recognition of the advantages of having higher-level and specialized training, mainly because of their added value for entering the world of work and the possibility of greater autonomy, including at an economic and social level, is motivational factors related to the search for and integration into higher education.

Some considerations on what entry (access) and attendance at higher education may represent for each student can contribute to enriching the reflection and analysis to be carried out, interrelating different factors (variables) and different actors.

An excerpt from the text by Garrido and Prada (2016), referring to higher education, to develop critical thinking on the subject.

> In the current context, higher education presents multiple challenges and is characterized by a high level of demand. Higher education institutions seek to respond, on the one hand, to the increasingly specific demands of the ever-changing labor market and, on the other hand, to the need to produce scientific knowledge. It is thus a context in which success is defined not only based on the grades obtained by students, but also by integration and adjustment to different people, activities and contexts. This multiplicity of roles requires the student to continuously develop and apply a set of skills. (Garrido & Prada, 2016, pp. 25–26)

It is undoubtedly at a particular stage in their lives that young people decide to apply and enrol in higher education, which confronts them with new realities, certainly demanding from an adaptive point of view. In this transition phase, changes are varied, implying the need for adjustments not only in the rhythms of daily life, personal, family, and social, but above all, at an internal level, both psychological and biological, with implications for health and well-being.

From Apprentice to Professional: Reflecting on Paths of Structuring Training

The training path from apprentice to professional is based on a variable period depending on the choices made by the students, during which various teaching and learning processes take place, essential to the transformations required to obtain professional training.

In addition to the wide range of knowledge defined for obtaining higher-level training, there is a set of skills (Ceitil, 2010) implicit in the learning necessary for the adequate performance of different roles.

> This multiplicity of roles requires the student to continuously develop and apply a set of skills. Some of these are more oriented towards promoting the learning of specific contents or procedures, others are more centered on self-development and relationships with peers and institutions. These skills share an important characteristic – their usefulness both in academic, professional, and personal life. (Garrido & Prada, 2016, pp. 25–26)

Young people/young adults in these circumstances are the main actors in the construction of their transformation, which will be better or not, depending on the value they attribute to it, and which drives them towards the achievement of their objectives, with the expectation of being effective in obtaining the positive results.

However, a set of other factors, internal and external, can also influence them in their development, and the relative 'weight' of each of them must be considered, as well as the multiple factors present simultaneously, when it is intended that evolve positively towards personal, social, and professional fulfillment.

In this regard, reflecting on the influence of health/mental health in high-level training processes, which require the student to mobilize physical and mental capacities and functions; as an example, the analysis carried out by a higher education teacher from the Madeira Region, an expert in health, is transcribed:

> 'Healthy Body and Mind' influence the 'High Level Training Processes', since: – They allow giving free course to the innate intellectual capacities and those acquired through the individual's intellectual training development, translating into technology – increasingly accessible to young people – the ability to carry it out. – They allow learning to use the technological instruments available for harmonic and balanced training, preventing human dysfunction, with family and social translation. – They ask Educational Institutions and Trainers to correctly apply training processes and monitor physical and intellectual development for different levels. (RHG, 2022)

The training processes that take place in HEIs are designed to respond to different needs and emerging challenges in today's societies, seeking to boost the development of science, and disseminating it for the benefit of humanity. However, despite those processes being thought and elaborated with delimited purposes and concrete methodologies, many of which are predefined, they must allow the trainees/students not only to learn to execute and reproduce what is taught to them, but also to be co-creators in a process of discovering new answers to new social realities, in a globalized, complex, and constantly changing world. The uncertainties are multiple, requiring the mobilization of diversified coping strategies to preserve mental health.

From the Primacy of the Technological Age to the Desirable Balance

The use of digital technologies is increasingly widespread in terms of application in different scientific and professional areas. In terms of higher education, the use of these technologies and tools has expanded, and teaching methods in e-learning and b-learning formats have become more relevant, as evidenced in the recent pandemic period due to SARS CoV 2, allow long-distance and rapid communication are an achievement without precedent in a globalized world. The sharing of knowledge through the formation of uni- and multiprofessional partnerships and work networks and between students from various knowledge centres and HEIs at national and international levels, are undoubtedly advantageous for the broadening and deepening of knowledge.

In this context, as an example, I would like to share an extract from a reflection carried out by another university professor, with specific training in technologies, on the following question: To what extent is the use of information technology an essential tool for learning and developing skills? Competences of higher education students nowadays?

He replied:

> We can divide the use of information technology into before and during the pandemic. Before the pandemic, it was an important tool, since its use allows access to new forms of interaction between students themselves and between students and the chair. This allows virtual meetings or asynchronous communication, allowing a better use of time and its distribution by the student. Likewise, in our case via B-On, students have access to a quantity and quality of bibliography unthinkable decades ago. And they can access, additionally, online tutorials on topics they wish to deepen or that are not taught in the disciplines. This makes the training paths much freer and not strictly linked to the contents of the curricular units. This last point is clearly evidenced in the variety of topics that are addressed in the master's theses. During the pandemic, all of this was enhanced, since remote access to both the university (classes, meetings with teachers and colleagues) and access to study material (bibliography, handouts), had to be done exclusively by technological means. (EF, 2021)

Since HEIs are responsible for preparing their students for successful integration into society, assuming different qualified roles essential to balanced development and global sustainability, they are inherently transforming contexts that must be at the forefront of innovation and scientific advancement, using resources for this to be possible. In the so-called era of the digital revolution (Magalhães, 2021), students, from the very beginning of their training, are called upon to develop skills that enable them to profitably use different technological tools, without mastering which they will not be able to integrate as professionals. For the transformation required in current times in the various productive sectors, including the vast array of health sectors, the challenge of developing skills asserts itself in the most varied dimensions associated with the need to invest in professional and digital training, whether at a personal or organizational level (Magalhães, 2021).

In parallel with all the technological evolution at a global level, educational innovation 'emerged' and 'imposed itself' with the integration of digital technologies. According to Arabit-García et al. (2021) professors, students, and communication media, constitute the classic triangle of didactic interaction. This new reality in which much of the communication can be privileged through digital means and channels, including the terms of training processes, spreads with some speed, demanding from the different actors of the educational and social contexts, specific training, and due consideration, regarding its impact on balanced development and mental health, in critical and structuring formative stages, both personally and for societies. Still, with reference to Arabit-García et al. (2021), in Europe, different models of analysis of the digital competence of teachers were developed, considering that the teacher, despite mastering the technical skills for the use of digital technologies, must also apply them in a pedagogical context. Students are considered digital natives or residents, mastering the use of technologies. As for the means of communication, they constitute a wide field of study due to the continuous development of technologies.

There are several advantages arising from the use of digital technologies and tools, however, there are also pertinent questions regarding inappropriate and excessive use, giving them full primacy in training processes, as well as issues associated with the improper manipulation of data, namely personal data, and organizational matters, without considering ethical and data protection principles and procedures.

Health/Mental Health Interconnections, The Use of Digital Technologies and Training Paths, as Pillars of Human Development and the Progress of Societies

Analyzing the interconnections is undoubtedly a necessary and simultaneously demanding task. The weighting of the advantages and possible disadvantages associated with the respective use raises interest not only on the part of students but also on the part of educators/trainers. The pedagogical experience places those involved in the teaching–learning processes in situations in which the use of digital technological tools is essential and useful, but it can also provide access to others, in which their use as disruptive or disruptive. By way of example, we mention that indiscriminate access to an extremely wide range of information, at any time, can create complex problems. Critical discernment is essential to create safer and healthier educational environments. It is essential, throughout the development, socialization, and training processes, to invest in the acquisition and reinforcement of literacy, whether digital or for the promotion and preservation of health in its various dimensions: bio-psycho-social and spiritual, or even for the safeguarding of human rights and the sustainability of face-to-face, affective, and socially structuring relationships.

The use of 'Information Technology and Training Paths' interacts with 'Health/Mental Health' and with 'Human Development and the Progress of Societies' in a positive and negative way. Let's see: 'Positive Points – Facilitates the reduction of interpersonal and socio-family asymmetries, reducing individual and group anxiety; and, consequently, facilitating interaction in training. – Expansion of means of measuring the applied methodologies, being able to obtain tools that can enhance the quality of teaching'. 'Negative Points – Difficulty in controlling bad technological practices, namely in computer-based assessment processes. – Reflection on security issues of knowledge bases (Cyberattacks). – Reflection on the security of the holders of knowledge. – Facilitation of personal isolation and lack of face-to-face/sensory interaction, which may trigger, aggravate and/or mask disturbances of bio-psycho-social origin'. Ultimately, it leads us to the obligation of comparing the results between the traditional face-to-face pedagogical methodology and the computerized methodology. Perhaps, the key question for an upcoming research project. (RHG, 2021)

The opportunity of these contributions for reflection is relevant. They reproduce a critical perspective that has been shared several times by different authors interested in the deeper study of the impact of technologies on styles and rhythms of life, both individual and community. The surrounding contexts, the pedagogical practices, and the applied teaching and assessment methodologies are essential to progress in the acquisition of knowledge, but also of new skills that allow personal fulfillment and affiliation and belonging to different groups and contexts. Throughout the life cycle, these needs are fundamental and significant from an intellectual and emotional point of view and have an impact on health and mental balance.

In this same perspective of using digital channels of communication/interaction in student training, another teacher noted:

These accesses, on the other hand, change the way in which students relate to their colleagues, friends, teachers, and surroundings. And it forces students to overcome an emotional/affective/psychic strength that is much stronger than that derived from face-to-face interactions. It is essential to monitor the mental health of students to accompany them in these challenges. (EF, 2021)

In the daily lives of those involved in higher education, time is dispersed and urgent for a set of essential activities and tasks regulated by norms, regulations, and established criteria, which aim to improve the quality of teaching and obtain the best classification results in the evaluative rankings. However, concomitantly, evidence has shown that other dimensions are significantly associated with learning and full and harmonious development. Welfare, health, and mental health stand out.

Initiatives and Projects Promoting Mental Health Literacy in HEIs

As far as mental health is concerned, there is currently more consensus on its relevance in various living environments, including academic ones, with the possibility of or even providing some psychological support to students (Portugal, Ministério da Saúde, Direção-Geral da Saúde, 2022; World Health Organization, 2021). The determinants of mental health (Lethinen, 2008; Moreira & Melo, 2000; Oliveira, 2020; Sequeira & Sampaio, 2020) are multiple and include a vast set of variables not only intrinsic to the person but also environmental and socio-cultural. Scientific evidence has shown that students' cognitive capacities, motivation, relationships with themselves and with peers, emotions, physical and sensory capacities, along with other constraints of the academic, family, and socio-cultural environment, such as, associated with pedagogical processes, that is, pedagogical relationship between students and teachers, and contribute to academic success and failure. With the lengthening of the formative processes that have occurred for many young people and young adults, different phases and circumstances have been identified, in which signs of restlessness and malaise are manifested with greater intensity in those, also existing, on the part of different intervenient. In academic life, initiatives to prevent, support, and, if possible, lessen more negative consequences or major disruptions in terms of health and mental health, which culminate in greater failure or even dropping out of studies. Faced with the possible diversity of situations identified and based on current scientific evidence, in the areas of both health promotion and the prevention of effective mental health problems, it is known that the interventions that have the best results should be carried out by transdisciplinary teams, that act in a cooperative and continuous way, in order to structure their projects, adapting them to the needs of the public they are intended for. It should be noted that the participation of students, teachers, and other non-teaching members of the academy is advantageous for the feasibility and acceptance of the various projects that may be implemented. In the country (Portugal) and inthe region (Madeira), there are examples of good practices in the implementation of projects that promote well-being and mental health, as well as preventive ones, whether they are universal, selective, or indicated (Gordon, 1987; Moreira & Melo, 2000) Notwithstanding, since these projects are initiatives to support mental health and well-being, it is ensured that any member of the academy decides autonomously whether or not he intends to participate and make his contributions to them.

Below are some notes regarding the development of projects of this nature, which can be considered for reflection and deepening:

- The opportunity and pertinence of the projects must be evaluated within the academic and student community itself if we want them to motivate their respective participation.
- The survey of expectations and needs must be combined between the various players.
- The prioritization of needs and identification of problems in the area of mental health must be carried out with the effective collaboration of professionals with sensitivity and specific training, after being validated with the public/ groups that want to be involved.

- A negotiable intervention plan should be structured between the participants regarding its implementation.
- Participatory and dynamic strategies and methodologies must be proposed for the respective implementation, which suit the characteristics of the participants, mobilize the available resources, which allow the achievement of the jointly defined objectives, and enable the achievement of results and gains in health/mental health.
- The results must be visible, after a joint evaluation of the implemented processes and considering the indicators selected for their evaluation.

The co-responsibility of the different actors is essential and the gains that come out should be positively highlighted, sharing how gratifying they can be among all.

Important aspects of the different interrelated stages were highlighted, which will be structural components of a collective work project, which is intended to be successful and with a positive impact on the well-being of academia (Project Management Institute, 2018).

Several focuses for interventions are possible, as well as different strategies and methodologies, including digital ones, with the primary aim of strengthening literacy in mental health and health (Knight, 2022; Sequeira et al., 2020; World Health Organization, 2010). The fact that this theme is included in the priority agenda of those responsible for the governance of academic contexts is certainly beneficial and fruitful for the pursuit of the strategic objectives of the educational community at the level of higher education, as it will contribute to making environments healthier, raising the good-being of the members of the academy, and providing them with different opportunities for the integral development of their abilities and personal, professional, and social fulfilment.

Trainees will not only spread in-depth knowledge but will use and make the most of their potential and skills, perceiving and feeling their mental health reinforced.

I end by quoting Simões et al. (2015), when he states:

> The superior performance of experts seems to be due, at least in part, to their ability to distinguish relevant information in a given context (p. 139), a statement to which I dare add that, for this, experts also need to know how to take care of their health/mental health. They can certainly become better 'equipped' during the training course carried out, for life in complex societies, but which want to be harmonious, balanced, developed and sustainable. (UN, 2015)

Final Reflection and Conclusions

The awareness that, at the end of this article, the theme whose approach was initiated needs further development and justification, both from a theoretical point of view and in the context of scientific research, which systematizes the study of the different variables that underlie and/or are associated with it, is expressed here.

However, the focus on it as well as the exploratory methodology adopted – sharing some questions with fellow higher education teachers from three different training and scientific areas – engineering, management, and health, as well as based on our pedagogical experience and human experience from academia, strengthen the assumption that we are facing changes, and transformations in HEIs, with implications for training processes and with influence on the health, mental health, and well-being of the different protagonists of academic life.

I encourage readers to think about one of the conclusions that was shared by one of the teachers who collaborated in this incipient reflection:

> In conclusion, there is no doubt that technologies enable an immersive and interactive experience, as well as a motivating one. However, it still needs some research and development. Technology will influence the current pedagogical model, accelerating and diversifying pedagogical experiences, far above the traditional model, implying fundamental changes in the dynamics of classes. (EL, 2021)

I would add that I reiterate my conviction of the opportunity and pertinence of a broader transdisciplinary debate in academia on the interconnections suggested in this article: between health/mental health, the use of digital technologies and training paths, as pillars of human development and the progress of societies.

Another conclusion is that combining technology with the reinforcement of motivation to learn, taking advantage of the advantages of its adequate and proportional use, encouraging development of important competences, contributing to find different methodologies and tools to intervene in the resolution of old and new problems, and allowing social and human evolution.

I also conclude, reiterating at the same time, the importance of dedicating more attention and spaces to training and academic contexts, which enable thinking together, in well-being and mental health, providing conditions that favour integral development, well-being, and achievement of expectations and objectives. By reinforcing these basic pillars, the different participants in academic life are given the opportunity to feel significant both in a personal level, among their peers, and in the academic community and society.

To all readers, my grateful thanks.

Active Learning

Suggested Teaching Assignments

If you attend higher education, try to know what projects are taking place at the institution to promote well-being and/or mental health and participate.

Take advantage of periods when you don't have school activities to communicate with your colleagues face-to-face. For example, take a walk outdoors or enjoy sharing a joint activity of mutual pleasure.

Use online communication only when it is not even possible to enjoy the benefits of face-to-face communication, such as looking and listening directly to your friend or colleague.

Share your positive emotions with those you appreciate and cherish, and trust that when you are sad or struggling it is also legitimate to share them because everyone experiences these situations a few times over time.

Web Search

https://orsmmadeira.uma.pt
https://felizmente.esenfc.pt/felizmente
https://cintesis.eu/pt/nursid
Literacia em saúde | Sociedade Portuguesa de Literacia em Saúde (splsportugal.pt)

Exercise of Self-knowledge

Think about how much time and importance you have devoted daily to taking care of your health and mental well-being.
Record a situation that you felt positive and rewarding at the end of each day.

References

Arabit-García, J., García-Tudela, P. A., & Prendes-Espinosa, M. P. (2021). Uso de tecnologías avanzadas para la educación científica. *Revista Iberoamericana de Educación, 87*(1), 173–194. https://doi.org/10.35362/rie8714591

Associação Académica da Universidade da Madeira (AAUMA). (2022). *Projeto Mentes Brilhantes.* https://amadeira.pt/2022/05/28/as-mentes-brilhantes/

Carette, L., De Schauwer, E., & Van Hove, G. (2018). "Everywhere we go, people seem to know": And knowledge construction of mental illness in higher education. *Social Inclusion, (Students With Disabilities in Higher Education),* 207–217. https://doi.org/10.17645/si.v6i4.1683

Ceitil, M. (2010). *Gestão e desenvolvimento de competências* (3rd ed.). Edições Sílabo.

Coordinating Council of Polytechnic Higher Institutes (CCISP). (2021). *Report health and well-being behaviors of polytechnic higher education students. A diagnosis from the students' perspective.* Estudos e Documentos | Conselho Coordenador dos Institutos Superiores Politécnicos (ccisp.pt).

Council Rectors of Portuguese Universities (CRUP). (2021). *Health and lifestyles in higher education in Portugal (ES+Saúde).* https://www.esmaissaude.pt/

Garrido, M. V., & Prada, M. (2016). *Manual de competências académicas. Da adaptação à universidade à excelência da vida académica.* Edições Sílabo.

Gordon, R. (1987). An operational classification of disease prevention. In J. A. Steinberg & M. M. Silverman (Eds.), *Preventing mental disorders: A research perspective* (pp. 20–26). National Institute of Mental Health.

JISC. (2020a). *Learning and teaching reimagined: A new dawn for higher education?* https://www.jisc.ac.uk/about

JISC. (2020b). *Student-and-staff-wellbeing-report 6. From fixes to foresight: Jisc and Emerge Education insights for universities and startups.* https://www.jisc.ac.uk/about

Knight, C. (2022). *A guide to looking about your mental health.* (About Clare Knight (news-medical.net)).

Lethinen, V. (Ed.). (2008). *Building up good mental health. Monitoring Mental Health Environments Project, co-funding by the European Union.* National Research and Development Centre for Welfare and Health.

Magalhães, T. (2021). *Transformação digital em saúde. Contributos para a mudança. Associação Portuguesa de Administradores Hospitalares.* Almedina.

Moreira, P., & Melo, A. (2000). *Saúde Mental. Do tratamento à prevenção.* Porto Editora.

Oliveira, P. (2020). Determinantes em Saúde Mental. In C. Sequeira & F. Sampaio (Coord.), *Enfermagem de Saúde Mental. Diagnósticos e Intervenções* (pp. 64–66). Lidel.

Organization of United Nations. (2015). *The Millennium Development Goals Report 2015.* United Nations (ONU).

Portugal, Ministério da Saúde, Direção-Geral da Saúde. (2022). *Plano Nacional de Saúde 2021–2030. Saúde Sustentável: De tod@s para tod@s.* Direção-Geral da Saúde.

Project Management Institute. (2018). *A guide to the project management body of knowledge* (6th ed.). ISBN 9781628253825

Royal College of Psychiatrists. (2020). *Mental health of higher education students, CR231.* Mental Health and Higher Education – Procurar (bing.com)

Royal College of Psychiatrists. (2011). *Mental health of students in higher education, CR166.* https://www.rcpsych.ac.uk/docs/default-source/improving-care/better-mh-policy/college-reports/collegereport-cr166.pdf?sfvrsn=d5fa2c24_4

Sequeira, C., Carvalho, J. C., Gonçalves, A., Nogueira, M. J., Luch-Canut, T., & Roldán-Merino, J. (2020). Levels of positive mental health in Portuguese and Spanish nursing students. *Journal of the American Psychiatric Nurses Association, 26*(5), 483–492. https://doi.org/:10.1177/1078390319851569

Sequeira, C., & Sampaio, F. (2020). *Enfermagem em Saúde Mental. Diagnósticos e Intervenções.* Lidel – Edições Técnicas, Lda. ISBN 978-989-752-413-4

Simões, E. (2015). Resolver problemas e tomar decisões. In J. G. das Neves, V. G. Margarida, & S. Eduardo (Eds), *Manual de Competências Pessoais, Interpessoais e Instrumentais* (3rd ed., pp. 117–144). Edições Sílabo.

Tabor, E., Patalay, P., & Bann, D. (2021). Mental health in higher education students and non students: Evidence from a nationally representative panel study. *Social Psychiatry and Psychiatric Epidemiology, 56*(5), 879–882. https://doi.org/10.1007/s00127-021-02032-w

University of Évora. (2022). *Mental health assessment of higher education students.* Comprehensive Health Research Centre. https://mental-health-of-university-st.uevora.pt/

University of Madeira, Psychology Service. (2022). *Projeto well-being UMa.* Ser UMa é BEM Estar na UMa. http://scp.uma.pt

World Health Organization. (2010). *mhGAP intervention guide for mental, neurological and substance use disorders in non-specialized helth settings.* World Heatlth Organization. ISBN 978-4-154806-9

World Health Organization. (2021). *Comprehensive mental health action plan 2013–2030.* World Health Organization. Retrieved October 5, 2022, from https://www.who.int/initiatives/mental-health-action-plan-2013-2030

World Health Organization. (2022). *World mental health report: Transforming mental health for all.* Retrieved October 5, 2022, from https://www.who.int/publications/i/item/9789240049338. ISBN 978-92-4-004933-8 (electronic version).

Zapata-Garibay, R., González-Fagoaga, J. E., Asadi-González, A. A., Martínez-Alvarado, J. R., Chavez-Baray, S. M., Plascencia-López, I., & González-Fagoaga, C. J. (2021). Mental health stressors in higher education instructors and students in Mexico during the emergency remote teaching implementation due to COVID-19. *Frontiers in Education, 6*(June), 1–12. https://doi.org/10.3389/feduc.2021.670400

Chapter 4

Digital Library in Hospital: The Case of Digital Neurotic Library to Achieve Better Health Literacy of Patients and Caregivers

Berta Maria Jesus Augusto, Carlos Manuel Santos Fernandes and Sérgio Filipe Silva Abrunheiro

Coimbra Hospital and University Centre (CHUC), Coimbra, Portugal

Abstract

Digital communication supports are a relevant resource for the promotion of citizens' health literacy. Aware of this reality, in the last quarter of 2019, health professionals of Inpatient Unit A of the Neurology Service of the Coimbra Hospital and University Centre designed the 'Digital Neuroteca', which consists of a digital repository with various educational materials in video format, e-books, pamphlets, manuals, infographics, and directories to websites that include credible information, and other content selected by the health team. The selection criteria consider the clarity and credibility of the information in various areas such as risk factors of neurological disease, strategies, and products to support self-care and available resources. Regarding more complex contents, there is a concern to transform them into information accessible to citizens in general. These contents are accessed by patients/caregivers through a tablet/computer, in the presence of the health professional, and can also be sent by email. We got positive results with an increase of satisfaction of those involved – patients, caregivers, and professionals. Health professionals and patients/caregivers reported high satisfaction with the use of this resource given the clarity of the contents, which facilitate understanding and meet their needs, recognizing this tool as an excellent complement to the process of health literacy promotion.

Keywords: Health literacy; digital information; empowerment; communication; neurological disease; digital communication

Technology-Enhanced Healthcare Education:
Transformative Learning for Patient-Centric Health, 47–55
doi:10.1108/978-1-83753-598-920231004

Introduction

The use of mobile digital technology in clinical practice is expanding continuously (Choi et al., 2019). We have witnessed a paradigm shift in the vision regarding the citizen's position in health systems. It is not intended to be a passive subject of care, but rather involved and co-responsible in health decision making throughout their life cycle. This paradigm is enshrined in the health policies in Portugal, reflected in the National Health Plan 2021–2030, the National Programme for Health Education, Literacy and Self-Care, the National Plan for Patient Safety 2021–2026, the Manual on Policies and Strategies for Quality of Health Care, among others. It will be crucial to maintain the focus on the promotion of health literacy among our citizens, always considering the individuality of the person, in a multisectoral, multidimensional, and integrated approach (Arriaga, 2019). Citizens with higher levels of health literacy can manage their health better, navigate the health system better, and evaluate the care they receive. This reality will lead to a more rational use of health services, for example, of emergency services, contributing to the sustainability of the whole system. Considering this reality, it is necessary to strengthen the strategies and resources to promote citizens' health literacy, their health and disease prevention, and, consequently, their well-being, as well as increasing the effectiveness and efficiency of health systems (Direção-Geral da Saúde, 2019). The Directorate-General for Health assessed the levels of Health Literacy of the Portuguese population between 2020 and 2021. The assessment was part of the Health Literacy Survey 2019 organized by the M-POHL consortium and taking place in 15 Member States of the European Region of the World Health Organization (WHO). The results identified a higher proportion of participants with high levels of health literacy (categories of sufficient and excellent) than with low levels of health literacy (categories of problematic or inadequate). The percentage of people classified with a sufficient level of health literacy was 65%, and 5% were found to have an excellent level. In contrast, 7.5% of people were classified with an inadequate level and 22% were classified with a problematic level. The results show a slight positive evolution when compared to previous studies developed in this area, however, they highlight the need to maintain the focus on the promotion of health literacy (Direção-Geral da Saúde, 2021). The M-PHOL study (2019–2021) also showed that the most difficult tasks identified about the citizen's action in relation to health were: General HL: judging different treatment options, protecting oneself from illness using information from the mass media; Navigational HL; Communicative HL: getting enough time from physicians, expressing personal views and preferences; Digital HL: judging the reliability of information, using information to solve a health problem (M-POHL, 2021, p. VII), among others.

The Pathway to Health Literacy: The Digital Communication

Health literacy is defined as 'the extent to which individuals have the ability to obtain, process, and understand basic health information to use services and make appropriate health decisions' (WHO, 1998), making it crucial that health professionals can empower citizens in skills promoting access, understanding, and use of health information. This will only happen if health professionals, in their various contexts of intervention (individual and collective), use an assertive, clear, and positive language, reducing miscommunication, if they involve the citizen in the whole care process, assuming themselves as a vehicle for reliable information, always validating the understanding and use of this information, with a view to adopting a healthy lifestyle. These professionals are also expected to facilitate the navigability of the health system (Arriaga, 2019). Several studies show health professionals as one of the credible sources of health information that the population uses and trust (Espanha et al., 2016).

The use of different pedagogical resources, such as audiovisual, media, and interactive tools (Brito, 2020) are strategies shown that they facilitate the transmission of information, the therapeutic adherence, and also facilitate understanding between health professionals and patients.

M-POHL (2021) also highlights that regarding digital health literacy, the emphasis must be on providing easily accessible, high quality, trustworthy, understandable, assessable, and applicable health information, as well as communication via digital sources should be increased (p. IX).

In view of the above facts and the importance currently assigned to digital communication supports the process of health literacy promotion, a group of health professionals from an inpatient and outpatient service of the Coimbra Hospital and University Centre, specifically the Inpatient Unit A and Day Hospital of the Neurology Service, designed the *Digital Media Library*. This tool arose according to the needs felt by health professionals in the process of promoting health literacy among citizens.

Neurological pathology often generates dependence on self-care, requiring the citizen to change his lifestyle and acquire a set of skills, aiming at an effective self-management process of his disease.

The new health condition requires a process of adaptation by the person, with the need to integrate a set of changes in his/her life. This process requires the awareness of these changes and their implications in the new health condition, as well as the need to incorporate a set of skills so that this adaptation process can be achieved.

The person's involvement in the therapeutic process is substantially dependent on the understanding that previous behaviours may have been incorrect and that a different behaviour will promote adaptation to the new health condition. For this to happen, it is determinant that the health professional assumes himself as the instigator of the citizen's motivation. Therefore, he/she must consider all the health determinants, whether they facilitate or hinder this process. These determinants may be of an external nature (education, socio-economic status, and community conditions) or internal nature (meanings, beliefs and attitudes, and level of preparation/knowledge) (Almeida, 2020; Martins, 2021; Nunes, 2019).

It is therefore necessary to empower the person through a facilitating intervention based on good health literacy practice and methodologies. Researchers, practitioners, and policy makers should therefore realize the importance of understanding and improving people's proficiency in using digital resources for managing disease and/or promoting their health by measuring Digital HL (M-POHL, 2021, p. XXII).

In this condition, the health professionals who coordinate this project felt the need to have an information support, accessible, which, through the support of the health professional, could complement the training process of the neurological patient and/or his informal caregiver. The project developed thinking about the ability of a patient caregiver with low digital health literacy but who should be able to make decisions in health.

Is Digital Therapeutic?

Choi et al. (2019) show evidence of the implications of digital therapeutics in four domains: cognition, speech and aphasia, motor, and vision. Choi et al. (2019) reinforce that those different forms of digital therapeutics, such as online platforms, virtual reality trainings, and iPad applications, have been investigated in many trials to test 'its feasibility in clinical use'.

Thus, in the last quarter of 2019, a digital repository was created that selectively integrated a set of clear, reliable, and targeted content to the specific needs of users of the neurology service, and aimed to respond to a problem identified by the project coordinators, namely the high quantity and diversity of information available on the internet that is highly complex and not very credible.

WHO Chief Scientist Soumya Swaminathan points out in WHO, Science in 5 (WHO, 2023), that she sees digital technologies expand, with more people having access to these tools, including healthcare professionals, thus allowing the latest information to reach people so they can take better care of their health (WHO, 2023).

Methodology for the Creation of the Digital Library: The Core Steps From Implementation to Evaluation

For the creation of the '*Digital* Neuroteletics', numerous *meetings* of the multidisciplinary team were held, using brainstorming technic, with the purpose of promoting the involvement and active participation of the whole team in the project. The team start to *identify the contents* to be included in the repository, defining the methodology of use, and defining the *project's assessment indicators*. This whole process was based on the assumptions and methodologies of *good health literacy practice* (Lopes & Vaz de Almeida, 2019). After collecting the various contributions, the leadership team systematized the entire project methodology in a procedure, which was disclosed to the team. At the same time, the preparation of the repository began, integrating the most *varied pedagogical resources* such as videos, images, e-books, infographics, manuals, pamphlets, and *flyers* that were appealing and presented simple and clear information, potentially understood by citizens in general. With more complex content, there is a concern to transform it into accessible information that is easier for its consumers to understand. *Pre-tests* were carried out before the implementation of this tool, involving patients and informal caregivers, to listen to them about the clarity of the contents. *Hyperlinks* were also attached to credible websites such as those of patient and caregiver associations and other community resources that may complement the information transmitted during inpatient/outpatient treatment. The selected contents were incorporated into a *set of categories*, namely: Pathologies; Self-care; Therapeutic regimen; Support products; Prevention of complications; and Caregiver and General information, suggested by the health professionals who make up the service team. Specifically, in this tool information can be found on: the various neurological pathologies most prevalent in the service (e.g., stroke, dementias, multiple sclerosis, amyotrophic lateral sclerosis, …); adaptive strategies and health support products for self-care (hygiene, dressing and undressing, eating, drinking, walking, positioning, transferring, and other); therapeutic regimen (healthy lifestyles, safe use of medication, strategies for adherence to the therapeutic regimen …); prevention of complications (pressure ulcers, fall, aspiration in dysphagia situation, ankylosis, infection, …); information for the informal caregiver (care techniques, available support and resources, promotion of their well-being, accessibility to support products such as articulated beds, wheelchairs, pressure relief devices, transfer devices, self-care devices, …); and miscellaneous general information (living will, status of the informal caregiver, citizens' rights and duties, contacts of patients' associations, navigability in the health system, accessibility to health services, *digital* support *apps*, …).

The implementation of the project included eight ($N = 8$) *training sessions*, with a total of 24 hours, on the use of good health literacy practices and the use of the digital repository, addressed to all health professionals in the service.

A *questionnaire* was applied to the professionals before and after the training session allowed us to verify that they had a limited understanding of the concept of health literacy and were unaware of a set of strategies and resources to promote health literacy.

To validate whether the person will know how to use the information transmitted, health professionals put forward *hypothetical situations* related to the person's health situation, appealing to the mobilization of the new skills acquired.

When appropriate, or by the request of patients or informal careers, the selected content is made available and send to their email and regularly updated.

The *continued spread of content useful* for the target is a process to which the entire multidisciplinary team contributes, under the coordination of the development team.

Clear and Positive Communication Is the Key: Supporting the Patient on the Digital Walk

This digital repository is accessible to all health professionals in the service who were timely trained in its use. In these training sessions, several communication strategies promoting the therapeutic relationship with the person were also reflected upon, such as the ACP model (assertiveness, clarity, and positivity) (Vaz de Almeida, 2021).

The importance of attending to the dimensions of access, understanding, and use of health information was also highlighted. The information content is made available to users using tablets acquired for this purpose and provided by health professionals (preferably by the reference professionals), who remain close to the patient and/or informal caregiver to clarify any doubts and validate their understanding.

Information is provided by the health professional in a selective and non-random way, based on the individual's needs and characteristics. Information is transmitted in a piecemeal manner, using the *chunk and check* strategy, repetition of content, primacy and recency, intentional questioning, deconstruction of numeracy, and always using an assertive, clear, and positive communication – ACP model (Almeida, 2019).

The access by the patient to the caregiver of the information, in the presence of the health professional, reinforces and consolidates the research, the assisted reading, and the comprehension. This process of proximity to the recipient allows the validation of understanding the information transmitted, for example, through the *teach-back* technique, giving the opportunity to clarify misinterpretations and synthesize the contents considered most relevant.

The 'Digital Neurotic Library' actually integrates contents prepared by the service's in the Hospital, based on good health literacy good practices.

To assess satisfaction with this project, opinion surveys are applied twice a year to health professionals and patients and/or informal caregivers who are the target of training. Health professionals expressed their satisfaction with the use of this resource due to the availability and easy access to different information adjusted to the needs of neurological patients, allowing for a more uniform message to the patient. Patients and/or informal caregivers were equally satisfied with

Table 4.1.   'Top 10' Categories and Subcategories Accessed.

Categoria/Subcategoria
Multiple sclerosis
Dietary regime
Support products
Medicinal regime
Stroke
Headache|migraine
HTA
Self-surveillance
General information
Caregiver support

Source: Own elaboration.

the diversity and clarity of the contents made available and their adequacy to their needs. Their expressions included: 'these videos allowed me to better understand how to lift my father … I didn't know there were so many products that help us in our daily life …'.

In 2022, this repository had 730 interactions by users, with an average interaction time of 10 minutes and 15 seconds. The months with the highest usage were February, April, and August.

Table 4.1 shows the top 10 categories and subcategories accessed.

Results Show Good Practice With the Self-prerception of Satisfaction

The health professionals expressed their satisfaction with the digital library, with the previous training, demonstrating the desire to change their intervention, and seeking the best results in this neurologic area of hospital care.

In short, we can say that the *Digital Neurotic Library* has proved to be extremely important for the promotion of health literacy of the person being cared for, the informal caregiver, and the health professionals themselves. These findings are corroborated by scientific evidence, which shows the diversity of communicational strategies as a promoter of health literacy. In the short term, we intend to integrate primary health care in tzjhmhis project, promoting continuity in the provision of contents as well as in their dissemination, enhancing the evaluation of the use of the information provided and their integration into their new health condition.

Active Learning

A 22-year-old patient was admitted due to numbness of the right lower limb and double vision with an evolution of one month. After complementary examinations, she was diagnosed with multiple sclerosis. She knew nothing about the disease. During hospitalization, she frequently uses the internet through her mobile phone, accessing information mainly from blogs and social networks. After consulting this information, she confides with her boyfriend that she will not take the medication prescribed by the health team, since she will only need a daily vitamin D supplement. At discharge, the health team only informs the user about the treatment to follow, without informing her about the way and the 'places' where she can consult credible and clear information about the disease.

- What action should the health team have taken to change the attitude verbalized by the user of non-adherence to the prescribed treatment, identifying the good health literacy practices to be used in this situation?
- Identify the possible advantages/disadvantages of information technology in the promotion of health literacy.

Url of Recommended Projects	
Biblioteca de Literacia em Saúde – SNS [Health Literacy Library – SNS]	https://biblioteca.sns.gov.pt/
SNS 24 – Área do Cidadão [SNS 24 – Citizen Area]	https://www.youtube.com/watch?v=furz8SbuU2U
Health Literacy Media	https://www.healthliteracy.media/
'Did you know that there are Universal Precautions in Health Literacy?'	AHRQ Health Literacy Universal Precautions Toolkit	Agency for Healthcare Research and Quality
AIIA project	Health Literacy	https://www.youtube.com/watch?v=ZE5mKiKqin0

References

Almeida, C. V. (2019). ACP health communication model: Communication skills at the heart of cross-cutting, holistic and practical health literacy. In C. Lopes & C. V. Almeida (Coords.), *Health literacy in practice* (pp. 43–52). Edições ISPA [ebook]. http://loja.ispa.pt/produto/literacia-em-saude-na-pratica

Almeida, C. V. (2020). Health literacy: An emerging challenge – Contributions to behaviour change. In C. V. Almeida (Coords.), *Health literacy, an emerging challenge – Contributions to behaviour change* (pp. 10–20). Gabinete de Comunicação, Informação e Relações-Públicas do Centro Hospitalar e Universitário de Coimbra [ebook]. https://www.chuc.min-saude.pt/media/Literacia_Saude/Literacia_em_Saude_-_Coletanea_de_Comunicacoes.pdf

Arriaga, M. T. (2019). Preface. Empowering health professionals for improved citizen health literacy. In C. Lopes & C. V. Almeida (Coords.), *Health literacy in practice* (pp. 11–15). Edições ISPA [ebook]. http://loja.ispa.pt/produto/literacia-em-saude-na-pratica

Brito, D. V. (2020). Design saves lives too – The hidden power of visual literacy. In C. V. Almeida (Coords.), *Health literacy, an emerging challenge – Contributions to behaviour change* (pp. 47–51). Gabinete de Comunicação, Informação e Relações Públicas do Centro Hospitalar e Universitário de Coimbra [ebook]. https://www.chuc.min-saude.pt/media/Literacia_Saude/Literacia_em_Saude_-_Coletanea_de_Comunicacoes.pdf

Choi, M. J., Kim, H., Nah, H.-W. & Kang, D-W. (2019). Digital therapeutics: Emerging new therapy for neurologic deficits after stroke. *Journal of Stroke, 21*(3), 242–258. https://doi.org/10.5853/jos.2019.01963

Direção-Geral da Saúde. (Ed.). (2019b). Manual de boas práticasliteracia em saúde: Capacitação dos profissionais de saúde. Lisboa: DGS.

Espanha, R., Ávila, P., & Mendes, R. M. (2016). *A literacia em saúde em Portugal.* Fundação Calouste Gulbenkian.

Lopes, C. A., & Almeida, C. V. (2019). Introdução. In C. Lopes & C. V. Almeida (Coords.), *Literacia em saúde na prática* (pp. 17–23). Edições ISPA. [ebook].

Martins, M. M. (2021). Informal caregiver reflecting on their identity. In C. V. Almeida (Coords.), *Literacia em saúde, um desafio emergente – O poder e a dimensão do cuidador informal* (pp. 35–44). Coimbra.

Nunes, J. M. (2019). Reflections of a family physician regarding the health literacy course: Models, strategies and intervention. In C. Lopes & C. V. Almeida (Coords.), *Health literacy in practice* (pp. 33–41). Edições ISPA [ebook]. http://loja.ispa.pt/produto/literacia-em-saude-na-pratica

The HLS19 Consortium of the WHO Action Network M-POHL. (2021). *International report on the methodology, results, and recommendations of the European Health Literacy Population Survey 2019–2021 (HLS19) of M-POHL*. Austrian National Public Health Institute.

Vaz de Almeida, C. (2021). Eureka: A proposal of a health communication model based on communication competences of the health professional! The Assertiveness, Clarity, and Positivity Model. In C. Belim & C. Vaz de Almeida (Eds.), *Health communication models and practices in interpersonal and media contexts: Emerging research and opportunities*. IGI Books. https://www.igi-global.com/chapter/eureka/286826; https://doi.org/10.4018/978-1-7998-4396-2

WHO. (2023). https://www.who.int/emergencies/diseases/novel-coronavirus-2019/media-resources/science-in-5/future-of-healthhttps://www.who.int/emergencies/diseases/novel-coronavirus-2019/media-resources/science-in-5/future-of-health

WHO. (1998). *Health promotion glossary*. Geneva: Author.

Chapter 5

The Importance of Therapeutic Education on Chronic Diseases: The Potential of Digital Education

Cristina Valadas[a] and Ana Matilde Cabral[b]

[a]*Endocrinologia, Hospital Beatriz Angelo, Loures, Portugal*
[b]*Consulta Externa, Hospital Beatriz Angelo, Loures, Portugal*

Abstract

We are currently experiencing, in western societies, a new reality in health systems, the emergence of an epidemic of chronic diseases, which test and raise new challenges to the health systems. This exponential increase in chronic diseases has not been accompanied by updated training of health professionals in this area. The chronic illness implies a bilateral relationship, of commitment and compromise for life, in which the involvement of the sick person must be the rule. The scope of therapeutic education (TE) is making the person autonomous and helping them to maintain or improve their quality of life. To treat patients with chronic disease, health professionals need to adapt their knowledge to their new role in the therapeutic relationship. As for the methodology, a participative observational methodology will be carried out with the training of health professionals who work in this area. It is a descriptive work based on studies and works published by the main schools working in this area, with emphasis on the School of Geneve. The purpose is to identify the problem of chronic diseases, the challenges that patients and health professionals face and how to build educational projects, exploring the use of educational tools, including digital technology.

Keywords: Therapeutic education; autonomy; empowerment; chronic disease; multidisciplinary team

Technology-Enhanced Healthcare Education:
Transformative Learning for Patient-Centric Health, 57–73
Copyright © 2024 by Cristina Valadas and Ana Matilde Cabral
Published under exclusive licence by Emerald Publishing Limited
doi:10.1108/978-1-83753-598-920231005

Introduction

In recent decades, changes in lifestyle in western societies, combined with increased life expectancy, have brought a new reality to health care, the emergence of a new 'silent' epidemic, the epidemic of chronic diseases, non-communicable. World Health Organization (WHO, 1998) already referred to the fact that about 80% of programmed medical consultations are related to chronic diseases.

This exponential increase in chronic diseases has not been accompanied by the updated training of health professionals in this area. Schools and universities continue to train their professionals to practice medicine in acute diseases, in which the doctor and other health professionals are the main actors, leaving the patient in a passive role. On the other hand, the relationship that is established between the health professional and his patient is punctual, limited in time, and is intended to be effective with gratifying results and recovery of well-being and health.

Chronic illness, on the other hand, confronts us with the renunciation of the immediate concept of cure and implies a bilateral relationship, of commitment and compromise for life, in which the involvement of the sick person must be the rule because it is with them and from them that solutions must be built and found. The person with a chronic illness must be an integral part of the health team, his educational needs must be identified, and tools and skills must be provided to make him more autonomous, with knowledge and decision-making capacity regarding the management of his illness.

This is the scope of therapeutic education, in which the role of patient education is recognized as a therapeutic action that making the person autonomous, making them more aware of their decisions and responsible for their treatment, and helping them to maintain or improve their quality of life.

To treat patients with chronic disease, health professionals need to adapt their knowledge to their new role in the therapeutic relationship, training and acquiring new relationship skills, which allow them to understand, treat, and monitor the person with chronic disease.

As for the methodology, a participative observational methodology will be carried out with the training of health professionals who work in this area. It is a descriptive work based on studies and works published by the main schools working in this area, with emphasis on the School of Geneve.

The purpose is to identify the problem of chronic diseases, the challenges that patients and health professionals face, and how to build educational projects, exploring the use of educational tools, including digital technology.

The Importance of TE on Chronic Diseases

Chronic disease is now all over the world and especially in westernized countries and Portugal is no exception, responsible for much morbidity and mortality, and this problem is expected to increase over the next few years (International Diabetes Federation (IDF), 2022). The increase in average life expectancy and western habits are behind this silent pandemic.

Before 2020, around 80% of medical consultations were due to chronic diseases and it is expected to be so. Chronic diseases are characterized by their duration and the appearance of possible sharpness and complications (Diabetes Education Study Group (DESG); Educação TerapÊutica na Diabetes, 2016; Éducation Thérapeutique du Patient (ETP); International Diabetes Federation (IDF), 2008; Ivernois & Gagnayre, 1995). Treating a person with chronic illness is to accompany them along their life path, and with it to find strategies for their treatment and support, motivation to combat setbacks and overcome difficulties, and above all, a path for them to fulfil their life path with quality.

To be effective in these projects, we must know how to work as a team, establishing partnerships with the people affected, working to increase their knowledge of their disease, stimulating their adherence to the proposed treatments, and, most importantly, increasing their autonomy in the daily management of the same and their decision-making capacity.

Therapeutic education is defined by **WHO** as a 'comprehensive' and global approach of the patient and his/her family that provides them with the necessary support and knowledge, to better know and integrate their pathology into their daily life (**WHO**, 1998, 2003).

In chronic disease, therapeutic education aims to make the patient more autonomous, more knowledgeable about his pathology, and aware of his/her fundamental role in its management, and to realize its essential contribution to reducing acute complications and the appearance of chronic complications, and above all learning to live with the disease to improve their quality of life and the effectiveness of their treatment.

Therapeutic education has as its main purpose, promoting quality of life, and is a process not based on the disease, but based on the future.

The person with chronic illness must regain control of his life, relearn hope, and regain the feeling of effectiveness, that is, to regain his role as an active citizen with goals and desires.

Therapeutic education should be oriented according to the specific needs of each patient, priorities of the same, their comorbidity, and taking into account the psychological and social vulnerabilities of the same (DESG; Educação TerapÊutica na Diabetes, 2016; ETP; IDF, 2008, 2022; Ivernois & Gagnayre, 1995; Roger, 1951).

Brief Notes on the History of Therapeutic Education

Therapeutic education, as we see it today, is born in 1921 with the discovery and the first insulin treatment (Grimaldi, 2017). A disease that was deadly to type 1 diabetes, it becomes a chronic disease, in which the patient and his family, need to learn how to manage the disease in all its complexity, and from the outing with the immediate need to learn how to inject insulin. A new chapter opened in the history of medicine with the need to transmit knowledge and skills to the patient, so that he could be held accountable for his treatment. The history of therapeutic education has always been intricately linked to the evolution and treatment of diabetes, due to the characteristics necessary for the treatment and daily management of this chronic disease.

In 1926, in Portugal, after the discovery of Insulin, Ernesto Roma aware of the need to educate patients and their families and share knowledge creates the Protective Association of Poor Diabetics, where the education of people with diabetes begins.

In 1941, Elliott Joslin, a Professor in Boston, publishes the first manual for general practitioners and patients. However, about 50 years were necessary to recognize the efficacy of therapeutic education. In 1972, Leona Miller, an American Doctor, published article in the *New England Journal of Medicine* shows that the benefit of an educational program for poor diabetics in Los Angeles, which allowed for reducing the number of hospitalizations per year (Grimaldi, 2017).

In 1975, Jean Philippe Assal created in Geneve a unit for the treatment and teaching of diabetes. It surrounds itself with a team of health professionals, with psychologists such as Anne Lacroix, and pedagogues, creating a team in which education is practised that aims at the active participation of the person with diabetes, as well as their autonomy.

In 1977, it is created within the European Association Study Diabetes (EASD) the DESG.

In 1998, the WHO recognizes and defines therapeutic education (WHO, 1998, 2003).

From the Diagnosis of Chronic Disease to the Need for Therapeutic Education

The diagnosis of a chronic disease is determinant in the life of a person and that of his family. The diagnosis carries with it a threat and above all the loss of the feeling of integrity. When confronted with this announcement the person has to assimilate that he is no longer healthy, feels vulnerable and dependent, and must start a process of mourning for the health he has lost (Giraudet, 2010).

On the other hand, it has to find meaning and move on and the need arises more or less urgent, depending on the pathology, to reformulate and adapt knowledge and acquire new knowledge.

The person who is faced with the onset of chronic disease will need to know his disease and his treatment and needs to acquire skills in the management of his disease in its daily aspects, adapting his knowledge and procedures according to his life.

An educational process begins, but educating is different from informing, and therapeutic education differs from the absolute concept of education. Therapeutic education aims at the patient acquiring and integrating acquired knowledge from his personal experience, developing skills and management, and decision skills in the sense of autonomy. Therapeutic education uses education as a therapeutic means with additional effects and enhancers of the usual therapies (American Diabetes Association (ADA), 2017, 2018; DESG; Educação TerapÊutica na Diabetes, 2016).

On the other hand, health technicians who treat and accompany the person with chronic disease, functioning as if in a 'mirror' with their patient, also have to learn to modify their learned and replicated behaviours in their formative pathways, which are generally directive and paternalistic behaviours, imported from the medicine of acute patients, where patients by the clinical situation have a passive and expectant role. In chronic disease, a partnership relationship must be established in which the patient is a partner in the management of his disease and is part of the team. This 'delegation' of powers of the doctor, is not easy or intuitive to do. Health professionals who have been prepared over the years to deal with acute disease, a model centred on the health professional himself, must acquire communication and relational skills that allow a person-centred approach to the disease, with a global understanding of the person, not only of the disease but of the person who has the disease in its psychosocial dimension. Therapeutic education implies the existence of health professionals with recognized training that allows them to assume their role as educators (ADA, 2018; Educação TerapÊutica na Diabetes, 2016; IDF, 2008, 2009).

Therapeutic education in chronic disease is teamwork focused on the person with chronic disease, in which the learning and the acquisition of skills necessary for autonomy are done within this team, with the patient having the fundamental role. In a continuous and adaptable way about the perceived needs of the patient, therapeutic education aims for the person with the disease to acquire the technical, social, and decision-making skills that allow not only healthy choices but also the person to carry out his life project and to know how to better use the health resources at his/her disposal. Therapeutic education will make the person autonomous, empowering him (ADA, 2017; Camarneiro, 2021; ETP; Huard, 2018; IDF, 2009).

The team should be constituted as a support network that accompanies and develops with the person and his family his learning process. It is up to the team, the identification needs, the positive reinforcement of appropriate attitudes in a continuous process of motivation, and the structure of an educational project that responds to the identified needs.

Therapeutic Education in Chronic Disease: Person-centred Interview; The Importance of Communication in Clinical Interviews

In chronic disease, the relationship that is established between the doctor and his patient is a relationship for life in which mutual trust is a fundamental factor. The patient is a complex Bio-Psycho-Social being and the way we apprehend all this complexity in its interaction with the disease is to practice a medicine centred on the person and not on the disease, and this is the basis of the whole process of therapeutic education. The clinical interview centred on the person is the key point of this interaction that allows the health team to know their patient, their motivations and difficulties, and to realize their educational needs. In the clinical interview, the way we communicate is decisive and health professionals who deal with chronic disease should be trained in conducting a clinical interview centred on the person with empathy, congruence, and absence of judgement (DESG; Ivernois & Gagnayre, 1995; Lacroix & Assal, 2003; Roger, 1951).

Building the Relationship-Environment

The environment in which the interview takes place makes all the difference. We must pay attention to what surrounds us when we want to foster an empathic relationship, of mutual trust, in which the person will expose himself not only with words but also with emotions. The environment should be comfortable, minimizing physical barriers, avoiding background noise, avoiding interruptions and interacting with the person, and limiting the records on the computer or written notes, so as not to interfere with the dialogue (ETP; Haute Autorité de Santé, 2007; IDF, 2009; Región Centro y Sudamérica, Federación Internacional de Diabetes).

Non-verbal Communication

In the clinical interview, communication does not only refer to the content of the message, it involves feelings and emotions that people transmit. In the interaction with the patient, our attitude as a health professional matter, and we should not forget that what we do not say, but we demonstrate, is perhaps the most perceptible and important (Roger, 1951).

Most of what we communicate, we do in a non-verbal way. And our gestures, facial expressions, posture, and behaviour will show the other our interest in him, our empathy, and our congruence between what we say and what we express. In the same way, our lack of congruence, the lack of interest shown in posture and gestures, can lead to a lack of confidence and the breaking of a relationship that is therapeutic. Put another way, it is impossible not to communicate, because non-verbal language is the most perceptible way to communicate.

The Person-centred Interview

All interviews and all dialogues necessarily have their dynamics and interactions. The objective of our interview in the course of a therapeutic education program is to use this relational dynamic to help the patient verbalization of their problems and needs as much as possible. The model used is often the person-centred interview, developed by Carl Rogers (1951). It is a non-directive interview, based on empathy, desire, and willingness to understand the person with whom we dialogue. The person-centred interview presupposes an attitude of interest in the other, availability and encouragement that predisposes the person to express himself authentically.

The doctor assumes an attitude of non-judgement, which allows listening and welcoming without criticism and guilt.

There must be a non-directive attitude, in the conduct of the interview, an attitude of openness, of encouraging the expression of problems by the other. In this kind of clinical interview, there is a genuine effort to penetrate the universe of the other, to understand it. In the relationship established between the doctor and the person, three attitudes of the therapist are distinguished and marked by Carl Rogers (1951) as facilitators:

Positive unconditional consideration: It involves accepting the person as they are and expressing positive consideration for them being as it is – Empathy:

Empathy consists of the ability to put ourselves in the place of the other, to see the world through his eyes, and to seek to feel what he feels. It is to have sensitivity to the needs, perceptions, attitudes, and emotions of the other. Empathy promotes the feeling of sharing with the other person (Roger, 1951).

One of the consequences of empathic understanding is the other feeling valued, cared for, and accepted as it is – Congruence:

Congruence: It has to do with the internal coherence of the therapist himself in his interaction with the other (Roger, 1951).

When we do an interview, we are communicating and communication has to be clear and effective. So, we have to make sure that we use a simple language, not a technical language, but rather appropriate at the socio-cultural level of the other person, taking into account that the cultural roots can be very different and that the same word can have very different meanings for each of the actors.

A communication technique must be trained in the so-called Active Listening, which is a communication technique, still based on the work of Carl Rogers. In their words of himself:

Active Listening means giving the other full attention and making him realize that we are interested and focused… Listening is a difficult job that you can only do if you have deep respect and care for the other.

We don't hear only with our ears but also with our eyes, the brain, the heart, and our imagination as well. More than hearing the words of the other, we perceive the message behind the words.

Highlighting the Practical Aspects in the Interview, Using Active Listening

The practice of Active Listening assumes that the therapist knows how to listen and he demonstrates to the other that he is listening to him. Some practical rules should be observed in Charts 5.1 and 5.2.

Chart 5.1. Learning to Listen.

- CONCENTRATE before each interview – create a calm, distraction-free environment
- OPEN MIND – be flexible, don't put yourself on the defensive, and avoid preconceived ideas
- Listen to the patient's point of view – think about him and not what you have to tell him
- Let the patient expose his thoughts WITHOUT INTERRUPTIONS
- If the patient interrupts LISTEN to him
- GIVE THE PATIENT TIME to answer the questions: do not interrupt the breaks
- TAKE ATTENTION TO THE ATTITUDES AND BEHAVIOURS OF THE PATIENT – these allow us to identify 'cues'/'clues'
- LISTEN TO THE VOICE OF THE PATIENT – the tone, the emphasis, the rhythm, and the silence are excellent indications of the patient's feelings and how he reacted to what he said.
- INTERCALE DEMONSTRATIVE EXPRESSIONS OF INTEREST – show that you are listening to it

---

Source: Own elaboration based on Carl Roger and Richard Farson (1957).

Chart 5.2. Steps for Active Listening.

---

1. KEEP EYE CONTACT: It is necessary to show the other that we are paying attention to him and not the other thing. This contact should not be intimidating
2. USE SILENCE: The use of silence is fundamental because it allows us to focus on what the other person says (whether verbally or non-verbally due to their attitude and gestures)
3. USE NON-VERBAL STATEMENTS: The use of non-verbal statements like smiling, waving, uhm uhm … etc., allows the other to feel heard
4. USE FACILITATION: Silence encourages answers and paraphrases what was said
5. USE OPEN QUESTIONS: Ex: 'So how have you felt?' Open questions allow the other to answer broadly and have the perception that they want to hear it and that it is
6. CLOSED QUESTIONS: When we want to get an objective answer, we have to use a closed question. For example, How old were you when your brother died?
7. CLARIFY: It is essential to leave no doubt that I knew what was meant to clarify when it is important.
8. USE THE REFORMULATION: Reframing what you were told allows you to verify the understanding of both sides (until then, one can only assume that one understood the other)

Chart 5.2.   (*Continued*)

9. USE THE SUMMARY: Repeat the main points of what was said to strengthen your understanding and show that you paid attention

10.   USE THE REFLEX: If the person shuts up and there is a pro-longed silence to the point of being a little at ease, one should simply repeat the last word or expression that has been said and wait

11.   USE VERBAL AND NON-VERBAL CUES: Do not forget that what you do not say is as or more important than what you're saying

Source: Own elaboration based on Carl Rogers.

A therapeutic education program comprises *four stages* described in Fig. 5.1.

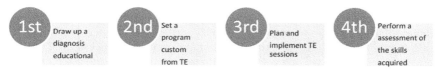

Fig. 5.1.   Stages of a Therapeutic Education Program. *Sources*: Vallier (2010), SPD (2018), and ETP.

1st Develop an Educational Diagnosis: Identification of Needs

Who is that person and how do you live with your illness?

To develop an educational program related to a patient and according to him, we must know that person in its many facets. Who is that person besides the disease he has? How is your interaction with the diagnosis of your chronic disease? After a chronic illness diagnosis, the person confronted with the news that will forever change his future must go through a process of loss (health) and reorganize to make the mourning (Ivernois & Gagnayre, 1995; Lacroix & Assal, 2003).

Therefore, we need to identify the phase of acceptance of the disease in which it is, to know how to adapt our attitude to help the person in their acceptance process.

The model of the 'States of acceptance of the disease' developed by A. Lacroix and J. P. Assal (Lacroix, 1998) is inspired by the model of Mourning, Freud, and Kubler-Ross, applied to chronic disease. The following are the steps described in Chart 5.3.

Chart 5.3.   States of Acceptance of the Disease.

– Denial
– Anger
– Negotiation
– Depression
– Acceptance

Source: Own elaboration.

These emotional steps are natural and sequential, and this process requires time. It should also be noted that acceptance is difficult, and the person can 'get stuck' in one of these steps, for example, staying in denial or depression, needing help to overcome.

In any case, these steps are not watertight and are often revisited, according to the evolution of life and the disease itself (e.g. if a complication arises).

The perception of the state of acceptance of the disease is very important in the educational process ,as we know motivation it is essential for change and if the person is in a phase of denial or anger ,have no motivation or desire to change, and ,if necessary we must help her to overcome this phase (Hunt, 2011; Ivernois & Gagnayre, 1995; Lacroix & Assal, 2003).

It is also important to determine the person with whom we are, how it works, what their usual pattern of adaptation to problems, especially tress, that is, their *adaptation or coping strategies* focused on the problem or centred on emotions (Lazarus & Folkman's Psychological Stress and Coping Theory, 1984) and whether that person has an internal/external control locus (Rotter, 1966–1975).

It should also be noted that the educational diagnosis is still essential to perceive that person, his willingness to treat himself, that is, only those who believe in the efficacy and cost/benefit of treatment can be accepted to treatment. This concept is addressed in the health beliefs model (Becker, 1974; Rosentock, 1988), which tells us about the perception of the disease and the perception of the severity of the disease, and, on the other hand, the perception of treatment benefits and the perception of obstacles to treatment.

All these aspects help us understand how that person usually reacts and how we can work with them towards their empowerment.

Pedagogical Approach in Patient Education

The 'systemic' approach to education is particularly useful when a patient is intended to acquire objectionable skills, such as therapeutic education.

The first stage is, therefore, the identification of the needs at that stage of their life and the path with the disease. Learning needs to change throughout your life as a person, throughout the illness and educational path, and therefore this needs assessment and it should be done whenever necessary (ETP; Hunt, 2011; Ivernois & Gagnayre, 1995; Lacroix & Assal, 2003; WHO, 1998).

The identification of the needs that is at the origin of the construction of an educational program will be done through the educational diagnosis, in which the pedagogical, psychosocial, and biomedical components are identified. Thus, the success of a person-centred educational program involves the correct identification of their needs and enhanced learning skills and motivation. It involves knowing, in that person, his illness and his evolution, but also his professional activity, family, social context, projects, conceptions and myths, the degree of acceptance of his disease, and learning potentialities.

Second, in the educational diagnosis, we should explore the different dimensions of the person concerned (Ivernois & Gagnayre, 1995; Lacroix & Assal, 2003):

- *Biological dimension* – What is it?
- *Socio-professional dimension* – What do you do?
- *Cognitive dimension* – What do you know?
- *Psychological dimension* – Who is it?
- *Dimension motivation* – What is your project?

At the end of this collection of information, we will be able to answer the question, who is that person, what is their understanding of their health situation, and what are their 'strengths' that may motivate the change and learning, but also identify their 'weaknesses' that can prevent or delay the process, which are urgent to identify to supplant.

The educational diagnosis should always be analyzed and discussed as a team and it will allow defining competencies to be acquired by that person, skills that are wanted relevant and realistic.

2nd The Personalized Program of Therapeutic Education

The program is based on the needs that are met during the educational diagnosis. The information collected allows you to better understand the person, measure their ability to manage the disease, and analyze their motivations. On the other hand, patients' perceptions about their ability or ineffectiveness are crucial factors to improve self-management and the results of treating their disease.

The person with chronic disease and the health technician agrees and define objectives to achieve, so-called learning objectives (Educação TerapÊutica na Diabetes, 2016; Lacroix & Assal, 2003; SPD, 2018; Vallier, 2010).

This commitment holds accountable and motivates the person with chronic disease to acquire skills and achieve the objectives defined together.

The development of a tailored program allows the person with chronic disease to commit to performing precise actions to become more autonomous in the management of their disease.

This process creates a positive learning environment and is the support to evaluate the success of the program.

3rd Plan and Implement Therapeutic Education Sessions

Educating is to train to develop skills and to optimize the skills and abilities of the person with chronic disease to accept and integrate change.

Participating in therapeutic education sessions is the best way for people with chronic diseases to acquire skills and achieve the abilities defined (Educação TerapÊutica na Diabetes, 2016; Lacroix & Assal, 2003; Simon et al., 2020; SPD, 2018; Vallier, 2010).

The sessions can be theoretical, informative, and/or practical, but should always be participatory.

Therapeutic education programs consist of individual education sessions and group education sessions that complement each other.

The type of session (individual or group) and frequency depends on the educational needs of the person with chronic disease and the resources available to acquire the pre-defined target competencies.

Any of them has pros and cons, and for this reason, we should make the most of the benefits of each type of session.

The individual education sessions allow a privileged relationship between the health technician and patient with the possibility of answering individual and specific needs, respecting the learning pace. This contact is more personalized and allows us to get insights about experiences from the patient, and in the end get a broader knowledge about it. This type of approach may become less structured, more repetitive, influenced by the health technician, and at risk of developing incompatibility, especially with more challenging patients (Lacroix & Assal, 2003).

The group and education sessions allow interaction between the various participants with an exchange of experiences. It becomes a more stimulating process in terms of learning with the confrontation of opinions and views. This approach allows it to work on various topics for a group of people with chronic diseases and thus save time. The difficulty of making all participants participate in the same way and heterogeneity is one of the main challenges. The health professional who is moderating these sessions may have difficulty managing the group and attracting everyone's attention. The stricter schedules of the programs and the risk of having a more directive and imposing intervention on the part of the health professional are risks that should be avoided (Lacroix & Assal, 2003).

Group training avoids repeating the same message several times, but it is necessary to use active/interactive methods to allow each participant to do the necessary learning. Today we are increasingly recognizing the advantages that group sessions offer, which allow stimulating and building different points of view. All meaningful learning operates based on previous knowledge. Pedagogy research insists on the need to provoke inter and intrapersonal cognitive conflicts. Numerous experiences in social psychology on behavioural changes show the benefits linked to small groups where participants can express themselves and show their points of view. It is easier for individuals to change their opinions and behaviours when participating in a small group. The health technician who manages the group should have a role as a change facilitator. These premises should be the basis for the construction of the different therapeutic education programs and in the development of tools to be used both in individual and group consultation (Lacroix & Assal, 2003).

Whether the therapeutic education program has individual consultations and/or group consultations, plans should be created based on each patient's individual preferences, values, and goals, and should take into account the patient's age, cognitive abilities, living conditions, health beliefs, support network, eating habits, physical activity, social and economic situation, complications and comorbidities, among others. This premise is not exclusive to this stage but should be present throughout the process.

4th Assessment of the Acquired Skills

The evaluation allows us to verify to what extent the person with chronic disease has achieved the expected learning objectives and acquired the required skills.

The evaluation should be made at all stages of the educational process as seen in Fig. 5.1. The evaluation in the different stages has different purposes, as you can see in Chart 5.4.

Chart 5.4.   Evaluation.

- In the educational diagnosis, to identify educational needs
- In the learning process, to adapt to the rhythm of the person with chronic disease and adjust to the difficulties felt
- At the end update the educational diagnosis, to monitor the ongoing changes, and make the necessary changes to the defined program

---

Sources: ETP, Lacroix and Assal (2003), Vallier (2010), and SPD (2018).

This evaluation allows monitoring of the experience and adaptation to chronic disease.

The review of the results of the management by the patient should happen without any accusation or judgements of value when 'non-compliant' or 'non-adherence' or when the results are not optimal. The family terms 'non-compliance' and 'non-adherence' designate a passive and obedient role for a person with chronic illness in 'following the orders of the health technician' who is in disagreement with the active role of people. An unjudgemental approach that normalizes lapses in self-management can help minimize patients' resistance to therapeutic plan adherence.

The objective of the therapeutic relationship is to establish a collaborative relationship (ETP; Lacroix & Assal, 2003; SPD, 2018; Vallier, 2010).

Tools for Therapeutic Education

The development of tools (traditional or digital) to be used in the education of the chronic patient (individual or group consultation) should allow the establishment of a dialogue and discussion with meaning, and in a logical way. It aims to inform, sensitize, and train participants about concepts related to their disease. Its development must be based on the Socratic approach, that is, questioning and discovery as a form to stimulate those involved to ask questions about their disease and to find their answers. The tool should be dynamic, stimulating participation, and with activities in which, individually or in groups, the final result is the result of the participants (Educação TerapÊutica na Diabetes, 2016; IDF, 2011; Lacroix & Assal, 2003; SPD, 2018).

These activities should encourage the involvement of participants in solving their problems and their contribution to solving the problems of others in group sessions, thereby increasing their knowledge and accountability. This is one of the appropriate ways in adult learning and it becomes fundamental when behaviour changes are needed to achieve greater therapeutic plan adherence (Batata et al., 2022; Camarneiro, 2021).

The forced isolation that the COVID-19 pandemic forced us to have an unavoidable way to bring digital tools into our daily lives. We learn that individually or in groups, it is possible to communicate, question, interact, and learn from a distance. Not replacing invaluable personal contact, digital allows on selected occasions, interaction, and facilitates the daily life of those who have and live with a chronic disease (ADA, 2022; Camarneiro, 2021; Región Centro y Sudamérica, Federación Internacional de Diabetes).

Conclusion

Chronic diseases now account for around 80% of our daily appointments. This 'silent' epidemic is a challenge for health systems, but also for health professionals, who work in this area, and who need more training in therapeutic education.

The appearance of a chronic disease forces the person with the disease to go through an adaptive process in order to rebuild his life with this new reality. The person with a chronic illness has to regain control of his life, relearn hope, and recover the feeling of effectiveness, that is to say, reassume his role as an active citizen with goals and desires.

Therapeutic education must be guided according to the specific needs of each patient, carried out by a trained team focused on the person with the disease, using the educational tools available, whether traditional or digital.

We strongly recommend five active learning sections at the end of the chapter (esta informação foi enviada num outro document):

1. Suggested teaching assignments (e.g. a list of 1–2 topics for short teaching assignment in the context of the chapter theme); for example, search the internet do two things or compile something and draft a report):

   - In chronic disease, when doing the clinical interview, for diagnosis, of the educational needs of the person with chronic disease, what attitudes of the health professional, which seem to him more facilitators of the clinical relationship?
   - What's the active listen for yourself?

2. Recommended readings (4–5 articles or videos publicly available for students):

   - http://archive-ouverte.unige.ch/unige:4125
   - http://archive-ouverte.unige.ch/unige:4126
   - https://www.betterconversation.co.uk/images/A_Better_Conversation_Resource_Guide.pdf
   - REF_aug2021_e20145_port (1).pdf

3. Case study (e.g. 1-page description – realistic: Something like two paragraphs description of a realistic real-world scenario and 2–3 questions for possible discussion):

Woman aged 60, born in Cape Verde but has been in Portugal for 30 years.
Married with 3 children, she works in an office cleaning company.
It has rotating hours (shifts from 4 p.m. to 12 a.m. and from 5 a.m. to 12 p.m.).
She has had type 2 diabetes mellitus for 15 years.
Therapy:
Metformin 850 mg 3× a day
Sitagliptin 100 mg 1× day
The family doctor referred her to the hospital's diabetes doctor because she had poorly controlled diabetes:

1. First appointment at the hospital:

   - You don't have blood glucose determination records (but you have a glucometer at home)
   - A1c – 10.4%
   - BMI – 38
   - Triglycerides – 186 mg/dl
   - Cholesterol –278 mg/dl

   A change in therapy was proposed:

1. Therapy change – liraglutide 1.5 mg weekly + insulin glargine 1× daily with fasting blood glucose measurement:

   - She was referred to the diabetes nursing consultation to start medication administration.

2. Second trip to the hospital nursing consultation – after 3 months:

   It presents lower blood glucose values with a loss of 6 kg of weight.

3. Third trip to the hospital for the medical appointment – after 6 months:

   - Shows weight gain of 6 kg.
   - Blood glucose values between 250 and 300 mg/dl.
   - What could have happened? How to find out?
   - What is the intervention of the health team?
   - How to overcome the situation?

4. Titles for research essays (indicative 3–4 titles for possible research works related to the theme of the paper):

   - The clinical interview at the time of diagnosis: Analysis of the testimonies of 10 adolescents with DM1.
   - Prepare a clinical interview to establish an educational diagnosis: the role of the multidisciplinary team.
   - What are the best tools to prepare health professionals for patient-centred interviews: interviews with health professionals.

5. Recommended Projects URL (indicative URLs from your current initiatives, professional):

- HAS – Haute Autorité de Santé: https://www.has-sante.fr/jcms/r_1496895
- Société européenne d'éducation thérapeutique du patient SETE: Site officiel de la SETE (Société d'Éducation Thérapeutique Européenne): socsete.org
- HUG – Hôpitaux Universitaire Geneève: https://www.hug.ch/en/patient-therapeutic-education-program
- Healthy Interaction: https://healthyinteractions.com/conversation-map-tools
- Language Matters: https://www.languagemattersdiabetes.com/
- Better Conversation Better Health: https://www.betterconversation.co.uk/; https://www.england.nhs.uk/blog/better-conversations-are-the-key-to-better-health/
- MS Pathways – Looking, Thinking and Acting Multiple Sclerosis: https://saudeonline.pt/nova-ferramenta-para-ajudar-doentes-com-esclerose-multipla/

References

American Diabetes Association (ADA). (2017). National Standards for diabetes self-management education and support 2017. *Diabetes Care, 40*(10), 1409–1419. https://doi.org/10.2337/dci17-0025

American Diabetes Association (ADA). (2018). Lifestyle management: Standards of medical care in Diabetes 2 – 2018. *Diabetes Care, 41*(Suppl. 1), S38–S50. https://doi.org/10.2337/dc18-S004

American Diabetes Association (ADA). (2022). Diabetes technology: Standards of care in diabetes – 2023. *Diabetes Care, 46*, S111–S127. https://doi.org/10.2337/dc23-S007

Batata, M., Braz, A., Camolas, J., Costa, A., Félix, I., Ferreira, H., Martins, H., Mendes, A., Nobre, J., Nascimento, D., Oliveira, C., Oliveira, M., Pimenta, N., Raimundo, E., Silva-Nunes, J., & Guerreiro, M. (2022). "Language Matters" Portugal: Recomendações sobre a Linguagem Preferencial na Comunicação Com e Sobre as Pessoas com Diabetes. *Revista Portuguesa de Diabetes, 17*, 26–33.

Becker, M. H. (1974). The Health Belief Model and Sick Role Behavior. *Health Education & Behavior, 2*(4). https://doi.org/10.1177/109019817400200407

Camarneiro, A. P. F. (2021). Adesão terapêutica: Contributos para a compreensão e intervenção. *Revista de Enfermagem Referência*, Serie V, Edição n° 7, 1–8.

Diabetes Education Study Group (DESG). Patient education. DESG Teaching Letter, No. 7. www.desg.org

Educação TerapÊutica na Diabetes. (2016). *APDP*. Scribd. [Internet]. https://pt.scribd.com/document/596688488/Educac-a-o-Terape-utica-na-Diabetes-2016Education Thérapeutique du Patient (ETP).*Haute Autorité de Santé*. [Internet]. https://www.has-sante.fr/jcms/c_1241714/fr/education-therapeutique-du-patient-etp

Giraudet, J.-S. (2010). *L'annonce diagnostique dans la maladie chronique*. Le Quintrec.

Grimaldi. (2017). Médecine des maladies. *Métaboliques, 11*(3), 307–318.

Haute Autorité de Santé. (2007). Éducation thérapeutique du patient Comment la proposer et la réaliser?*Recommandations*.

Huard, P. (2018). *The management of chronic diseases: Organizational innovation and efficiency*. John Wiley & Sons Incorporated.

Hunt, J. (2011). Motivational interviewing, and people with diabetes. *European Diabetes Nursing, 8*(2), 68–73b

International Diabetes Federation (IDF). (2008). *International curriculum for diabetes health professional education*. IDF.

International Diabetes Federation (IDF). (2009). *International standards for diabetes education* (3rd ed.). IDF.

International Diabetes Federation (IDF). (2011). *Peer leader manual*. IDF.

International Diabetes Federation (IDF). (2022). *IDF Atlas 2022* (10th ed.). IDF.

Ivernois, J., & Gagnayre, R. (1995). *Apprendre à éduquer le patient*. Éditions Vigot.

Lacroix, A., & Assal, J. P. (2003). *L'Education thérapeutique des patients*. Éditions Vigot.

L'Éducation thérapeutique des patients Anne Lacroix et Jean-Philippe Assal, Paris, Vigot, 1998

Región Centro y Sudamérica, Federación Internacional de Diabetes. (2022, August 5). *Guía de Práctica Clínica de Educación en Diabetes*. https://idfsaca.com/wp-content/uploads/2022/08/guia-de-practica-clinica-de-educacion-en-diabetes-en-idioma-espanol.pdf.saca

Roger, C. (1951). *Client-centered therapy: Its current practice, implications and theory*. Constab.

Rogers, C. R., & Farson, R. E. (1957). *Active listening*. Chicago, IL: Industrial Relations Center of the University of Chicago.

Rosenstock, I. M., Stretcher, V. J., Becker, M. H. (1988). Social learning theory and the Health Belief Model. *Health Educ Q*, 15(2), 175–183.

Rotter, J. B. (1966). Generalized expectancies for internal versus external control of reinforcement. *Psychological Monographs*, *80*(1), 1–28.

Simon, D., Bourdillon, F., Gagnayre, R., & Grimaldi, A. (2020). *Éducation thérapeutique: prévention et maladies chroniques*. Elsevier Masson.

SPD. (2018). *Educação Terapêutica na Diabetes: Competências dos profissionais de saúde e das pessoas com Diabetes*. Um Guia para Profissionais de Saúde. [Internet]. https://spd.pt/images/booklet_educacao_terapeutica.pdf

Vallier, V. (2010). *L'integration de la Maladie Chronique en Diabetologie: Apport de l'Education Thérapeutique au Patient*. Institut de Formation en Soins Infirmiers Nancy-Brabois.

WHO. (1998). *Therapeutic patient education: Continuing education programs for healthcare providers in the field of prevention of chronic diseases: Report of a Working Group*. WHO.

World Health Organization. (2003). *Adherence to long term therapies – Evidence for action* (pp. 1–85). World Health Organization.

Chapter 6

Health Literacy and Diabetes: Challenges and Trends

Dulce Nascimento do Ó[a,b], Ana Rita Goes[b], João Filipe Raposo[a,c] and Isabel Loureiro[b]

[a]*APDP – Diabetes Portugal, Lisboa, Portugal*
[b]*NOVA National School of Public Health, Public Health Research Centre, Comprehensive Health Research Center, CHRC, NOVA University Lisbon, Lisbon, Portugal*
[c]*CEDOC – Center for the Study of Chronic Disease, NOVA Medical School, Lisboa, Portugal*

Abstract

Diabetes is a chronic and challenging disease and requires personal daily self-management decisions and skills. For that, it is necessary that patients have sufficient information and health literacy to make the right choices and decisions in their self-care. Sequentially, health literacy has great relevance and influence in the daily lives of people with diabetes, since it encompasses the necessary skills to manage disease and health. Health literacy can be a relevant factor to consider when tackling diabetes self-management. Thus, for the prevention and treatment of diabetes, it is essential to promote individual health literacy. The quality of communication and patient-centred communication style seems to be a key aspect for the health literacy.

Keywords: Health literacy; diabetes; self-management; communication; person-centred collaborative care; chronic diseases

Introduction

Diabetes control is largely dependent on personal self-management, which demands individuals to perform a complex set of activities, including monitoring glucose, taking medication, eating a healthy diet, making regular physical activity, and constantly adjusting treatment to the condition status. For that, it is

Technology-Enhanced Healthcare Education:
Transformative Learning for Patient-Centric Health, 75–82
Copyright © 2024 by Dulce Nascimento do Ó, Ana Rita Goes, João Filipe Raposo and Isabel Loureiro
Published under exclusive licence by Emerald Publishing Limited
doi:10.1108/978-1-83753-598-920231006

necessary that patients have sufficient information, the necessary skills, and a facilitating environment to make the right choices and decisions in their self-care. Several studies highlight the importance of health literacy, related with better diabetes knowledge, metabolic control, and better communication with healthcare providers. Health literacy is also essential for community participation in health issues and planning. Therefore, health literacy can be a relevant factor to consider when tackling the impact of health outcomes. In this chapter, we will present available evidence related to health literacy and diabetes outcomes and discuss the challenges and trends in promoting health literacy within diabetes care.

Is Health Literacy Important for Diabetes Control?

Diabetes is one of the major health emergencies of the twenty-first century due to its increasing incidence and prevalence worldwide. There were an estimated 537 million people with diabetes in 2015, equivalent to one person with diabetes in every 11 people. By the year 2040, this is expected to increase to 643 million people with diabetes and 784 million by 2045, corresponding to one person with diabetes in every 10 people (International Diabetes Federation (IDF), 2021). In Portugal, the estimated prevalence in the population aged between 20 and 79 years in 2018 was 13.6%, that is, more than 1 million Portuguese in this age group have diabetes (Sociedade Portuguesa de Diabetologia (SPD)). This represents a serious problem because diabetes and its complications are the leading causes of early death in most countries. In 2021, it is estimated that 6.7 million adults aged 20–79 years will die from diabetes (International Diabetes Federation (IDF), 2021).

As scientific evidence has shown (American Diabetes Association (ADA), 2020) that it is possible to reduce the damage associated with this pathology through rigorous control of hyperglycaemia and other risk factors, like hypertension and dyslipidaemia. Adequately controlled diabetes means having blood sugar levels within personalized target limits. Despite the emergence of innovative drugs and technology for its treatment, there seems to be consensus in the scientific community that effective self-management and psychological well-being are essential to achieving treatment goals for people with diabetes (International Diabetes Federation (IDF), 2021; Powers et al., 2020).

Health literacy was defined by the World Health Organization as 'the cognitive and social skills which determine the motivation and the ability of individuals to gain access to, understand and use information in ways which promote and maintain good health' (World Health Organization (WHO), 1998). Health literacy is highly relevant in the lives of patients, families, and communities, involving many fields, from individual patient care to community-level development, from improving compliance to empowering individuals and communities, and for participation in community debates and planning about issues that affect health (Batterham et al., 2016). Beyond the importance for each person, health literacy is essential for health organizations' capacity to provide quality health care, and for society to ensure the health and well-being of its citizens (Sorensen, 2019). Therefore, health literacy is considered to be a relevant factor to reduce the impact of social disparities on health outcomes (Dodson et al., 2015; Okan et al., 2019; Osborn et al., 2011).

At an individual level, health literacy affects the ability to access, understand, remember, and use information, to access the increasingly complex healthcare system, as well as to deal with aspects related with prevention, health promotion and treatment of diseases, communication with others about health messages, and to make informed, conscious decisions about life and health outcomes (Dodson et al., 2015; Osborn et al., 2011). People with lower levels of health literacy may have difficulties understanding health information, what they read or what is communicated to them in consultations, which reduces their autonomy in self-care and decision making (Edwards et al., 2012; Erlen, 2004). Also, lower health literacy is associated with poor health outcomes, less healthy behaviours and lifestyle, and greater difficulty in developing self-management skills (Berkman et al., 2011; Sørensen et al., 2015). This situation is even more concerning in the older and less educated people because they tend to have lower health literacy (Marciano et al., 2019; Schillinger et al., 2002), are more susceptible to impaired health (Baker et al., 2000) and 'suffer most of the burden of inadequate health literacy-adverse health outcomes' (Toci et al., 2015). Given the demand for diabetes self-management and the importance of achieving good metabolic control, several studies have been developed to understand the impact of health literacy on diabetes outcomes. Accordingly, health literacy is related with better diabetes knowledge (Al Sayah et al., 2013; Bailey et al., 2014), better metabolic control (Gao et al., 2013), self-perceived better health (Bennett et al., 2009; Jovic-Vranes et al., 2009), and self-care diabetes (Marciano et al., 2019). People with type 2 diabetes with lower health literacy were two times more likely to have limited glycaemic management, with an A1C of 9.5% or greater (Schillinger et al., 2002). Also, higher levels of health literacy were associated with better communication between users and physicians, at higher levels of confidence (Al Sayah et al., 2013), while people with lower health literacy levels were more likely to report poorer communication with healthcare professionals (Bailey et al., 2014), and to be less willing to participate in the process of clinical decision (Boren, 2009). In other studies, an association between health literacy and diabetes compensation was found to be indirect and mediated by knowledge about diabetes (Bailey et al., 2014) or by social support (Osborn et al., 2010). For Lee and his collaborators, health literacy is associated with self-efficacy, which in turn is associated with self-care in diabetes, associated with diabetes compensation (Gao et al., 2013). This is also in accordance with theoretical models that propose health literacy to be an antecedent of health outcomes (Paasche-Orlow & Wolf, 2007), although some studies were not able to find such association between health literacy and diabetes outcomes (Caruso et al., 2018; Kim et al., 2004; Morris et al., 2006).

These different results may be explained by the use of diverse measurements of health literacy, usually focused on functional health literacy rather than on the skills needed to manage diabetes (Olesen et al., 2017). Nonetheless, when we consider health literacy beyond reading, writing, and math skills, to include social and communication skills that enable the use of health information and empower the person to participate in their care (Estacio, 2013), the importance of health literacy in the self-management of diabetes seems evident.

How to Improve Health Literacy in Health Care?

The identification of aspects that contribute for the improvement of health literacy in health care is quite relevant. One of the factors that seems to be a key factor in health literacy is the quality of communication (Sørensen et al., 2012). The communication strategies that health professionals use can lead to improved health literacy if they are relevant to the needs and interests and applied with an empowering approach (Almeida & Belim, 2019). Several policy documents and position statements recommend the use of 'teach-back' as a health literacy-based communication approach (Talevski et al., 2020). This communication strategy involves asking patients to explain in their own words what has just been told them. If needed, the healthcare provider clarifies any misunderstandings, and the understanding is rechecked. This process ends when the patient correctly reproduces the information that was given. The use of this technique has been shown to improve knowledge, skills, and self-care abilities in patients with chronic diseases (Ha Dinh et al., 2016; Negarandeh et al., 2013).

In this sense, and as expected, a clear patient–provider communication has a positive effect on diabetes outcomes (Talevski et al., 2020). In this regard, language, as the principal instrument for sharing knowledge and understanding, can have a strong impact on perceptions, motivation, behaviours, and outcomes (Dickinson et al., 2017; Dunning et al., 2017). The ADA Consensus (2017) suggests use of language that

> is neutral, non-judgmental, and based on facts, actions, or physiology/biology; is free from stigma; is strengths based, respectful, inclusive, and imparts hope; fosters collaboration between patients and providers; is person centered. (Dickinson et al., 2017)

Clear communication avoids creating barriers between patients and healthcare providers. Plain language defined as 'concise, well-organized, and follows other best practices appropriate to the subject or field and intended audience' is considered an important tool for tackling literacy barriers and improving patient comprehension (Centers of Disease Control and Prevention (CDC), n.d.).

Simultaneously, patient-centred communication style that 'uses active listening, elicits patient preferences and beliefs, and assesses literacy, numeracy, and potential barriers to care (...) optimize patient health outcomes and health-related quality of life', is recommended in several positions statement, including from the ADA and the European Association for the Study of Diabetes (EASD). This person-centred collaborative care is guided by shared decision making in treatment regimen selection and monitoring of agreed-upon regimen and lifestyle (International Diabetes Federation (IDF), 2021; Hill-Briggs, 2003).

This type of relationship appears as a new challenge in which health professionals need not only biomedical knowledge and competencies, but also pedagogical and relational skills, which promote the motivation, knowledge, and health literacy in people with diabetes to take responsibility and manage their treatment, knowledge, and health literacy (Assal, 1999; Sørensen et al., 2012).

Conclusion

In conclusion, the need for an emphasis on the promotion of health literacy in diabetes care becomes evident. Additionally, it also represents a challenge, because health professionals need specific health literacy competencies in order to respond to the needs of people with limited health literacy and improve person-centred care. Despite the recommendations to use the 'teach-back' and patient-centred approach (Bodegård et al., 2020), its use is not yet consistent. This may, in part, be related to organizational and interpersonal barriers, including lack of time, patient, and doctor's schedule, limited support by senior staff, and the need to develop communication skills. It also becomes more difficult for professionals to develop competencies in health literacy and patient-centered communication if this is not considered a priority in their team or organization, especially when time and allocated resources are limited (Kaper, 2021).

In this way, a more responsive healthcare system, and the training of healthcare providers to promote patient's health literacy, represent an important challenge and a needed trend *to leave no one behind.*

Some Relevant Websites

APDP-Diabetes Portugal: https://www.apdp.pt
National School of Public Health: https://www.ensp.unl.pt
Portuguese Society of Diabetology: https://www.spd.pt
International Diabetes Federation: https://idf.org/
American Association Diabetes: https://diabetesjournals.org/care

Recommended Readings

Manual of Therapeutic Education in Diabetes – SPD: https://spd.pt/images/booklet_educacao_terapeutica.pdf

Articles

Nascimento do Ó, D., Goes, A. R., Elsworth, G., Raposo, J. F., Loureiro, I., & Osborne, R. H. (2022). Cultural adaptation and validity testing of the Portuguese Version of the Health Literacy Questionnaire (HLQ). *International Journal of Environmental Research and Public Health, 19*(11), 64–65. https://doi.org/10.3390/ijerph19116465; https://pubmed.ncbi.nlm.nih.gov/35682052/

Nascimento do Ó, D., Serrabulho, L., Ribeiro, R. T., Silva, S., Covinhas, A., Afonso, M. J., Boavida, J. M., & Raposo, J. F. (2022). Interpersonal relationships in diabetes: Views and experience of people with diabetes, informal carers, and healthcare professionals in Portugal. *Acta Medica Portuguesa, 35*(10), 729–737. https://pubmed.ncbi.nlm.nih.gov/35239472/

Standards of Medical Care in Diabetes 2023, ADA: https://diabetesjournals.org/care/issue/46/Supplement_1

References

Al Sayah, F., Majumdar, S., Williams, B., Robertson, S., & Johnson, J. (2013). Health literacy and health outcomes in diabetes: A systematic review. *Journal of General Internal Medicine, 28*(3), 444–452. https://doi.org/10.1007/s11606-012-2241-z

Almeida, C. V., & Belim, C. (2019). Health literacy and health professionals: Open the door of communication for better outcomes. *Archives of Biomedical Engineering & Biotechnology, 2*(5). https://doi.org/10.33552/ABEB.2019.02.000548

American Diabetes Association (ADA). (2017, January). Standards of Medical Care in Diabetes 2017. *Diabetes Care, 40*(Suppl. 1), S4–S128. doi: 10.2337/dc17-S001.

American Diabetes Association (ADA). (2020, January). *Standards of Medical Care in Diabetes 2021* (p. 44). https://doi.org/10.2337/dc21-in01

Assal, J. P. (1999). WHO – Report on therapeutic patient education. *Medicographia, 21*, 4.

Bailey, S., Brega, A., Crutchfield, T. M., Elasy, T., Herr, Crutchfield, T., Elasy, T., Herr, H., Kaphingst, K., Karter, A., Moreland-Russel, S., Osborn, C., Pignone, M., Rothman, R., & Schillinger, D. (2014). Update on health literacy and diabetes. *Diabetes Education, 40*(5), 581–604. https://doi.org/10.1177/0145721714540220

Baker, D. W., Gazmararian, J. A., Sudano, J., & Patterson, M. (2000). The association between age and health literacy among elderly persons. *The Journals of Gerontology Series B: Psychological Sciences and Social Sciences, 55*, S368–S374.

Batterham, R., Hawkins, M., Collins, P., Buchbinder, R., & Osborne, R. (2016). Health literacy: Applying current concepts to improve health services and reduce health inequalities. *Public Health, 132*, 3–12. https://doi.org/10.1016/j.puhe.2016.01.001

Bennett, I. M., Chen, J., Soroui, J. S., & White, S. (2009). The contribution of health literacy to disparities in self-rated health status and preventive health behaviors in older adults. *Annals of Family Medicine, 7*, 204–211.

Berkman, N. D., Sheridan, S. L., Donahue, K. E., Halpern, D. J., & Crotty, K. (2011, July). Low health literacy and health outcomes: An updated systematic review. *Annals of Internal Medicine, 155*(2), 97–107. https://doi.org/10.7326/0003-4819-155-2-201107190-00005. PMID: 21768583

Bodegård, H., Helgesson, G., Juth, N., Olsson, D., & Lynøe, N. (2020). Challenges to patient centredness – A comparison of patient and doctor experiences from primary care. *BMC Family Practice, 20*, 83.

Boren, S. (2009). A review of health literacy and diabetes: Opportunities for technology. *Journal of Diabetes Science and Technology*. https://doi.org/10.1177/193229680900300124

Caruso, R., Magon, A., Baroni, I., Dellafiore, F., Arrigoni, C., Pittella, F., & Ausili, D. (2018). Health literacy in type 2 diabetes patients: A systematic review of systematic reviews. *Acta Diabetologica, 55*(1), 1–12. https://doi.org/10.1007/s00592-017-1071-1

Centers of Disease Control and Prevention (CDC). (n.d.). https://www.cdc.gov/healthliteracy/developmaterials/plainlanguage.html

Dickinson, J. K., Guzman, S. J., Maryniuk, M. D., O'Brian, C. A., Kadohiro, J. K., Jackson, R. A., D'Hondt, N., Montgomery, B., Close, K. L., & Funnell, M. M. (2017). The use of language in diabetes care and education. *Diabetes Care, 40*(12), 1790–1799. https://doi.org/10.2337/dci17-0041

Dodson, S., Good, S., & Osborne, R. (2015). *Health literacy toolkit for low and middle-income countries: A series of information sheets to empower communities and strengthen health systems.* World Health Organization, Regional Office for South-East Asia.

Dunning, T., Speight, J., & Bennett, C. (2017). Language, the "diabetes restricted code/dialect," and what it means for people with diabetes and clinicians. *The Diabetes Educator, 43*(1), 18–26. https://doi.org/10.1177/0145721716683449

Edwards, M., Wood, F., Davies, M., & Edwards, A. (2012). The development of health literacy in patients with a long-term health condition: The health literacy pathway model. *BMC Public Health, 130*. https://doi.org/10.1186/1471-2458-12-130

Erlen, J. (2004). Functional health illiteracy. Ethical concerns. *Orthopedic Nursing*, *2*, 150–153. https://doi.org/10.1097/00006416-200403000-00015

Estacio, E. V. (2013). Health literacy and community empowerment: It is more than just reading, writing and counting. *Journal of Health Psychology*, *18*(8), 1056–1068. https://doi.org/10.1177/1359105312470126

Gao, J., Wang, J., Zheng, P., Haardörfer, R., Kegler, M., Zhu, Y., & Fu, H. (2013). Effects of self-care, self-efficacy, social support on glycemic control in adults with type 2 diabetes. *BMC Family Practice*, *14*(66). https://doi.org/10.1186/1471-2296-14

Ha Dinh, T. T., Bonner, A., Clark, R., Ramsbotham, J., & Hines, S. (2016). The effectiveness of the teach-back method on adherence and self-management in health education for people with chronic disease: A systematic review. *JBI Database of Systematic Reviews and Implementation Reports*, *14*(1), 210–247. https://doi.org/10.11124/jbisrir-2016-2296

Hill-Briggs, F. (2003). Problem solving in diabetes self-management: A model of chronic illness self-management behavior. *Annals of Behavioral Medicine*, *25*, 182–193. https://doi.org/10.1207/S15324796ABM2503_04

International Diabetes Federation (IDF). (2021). *IDF Diabetes Atlas* (10th ed.). https://diabetesatlas.org/atlas/tenth-edition/

Jovic-Vranes, A., Bjegovic-Mikanovic, V., & Marinkovic, J. (2009). Functional health literacy among primary health-care patients: Data from the Belgrade pilot study. *Journal of Public Health (Oxford Journals)*, *31*, 490–495.

Kaper, M. (2021). *Improving communication in healthcare for patients with low health literacy: Building competencies of health professionals and shifting towards health literacy friendly organizations*. University of Groningen. https://doi.org/10.33612/diss.172455932

Kim, S., Love, F., Quistberg, D. A., & Shea, J. A. (2004). Association of health literacy with self-management behavior in patients with diabetes. *Diabetes Care*, *27*(12), 2980–2982. https://doi.org/10.2337/diacare.27.12.2980

Marciano, L., Camerini, A. L., & Schulz, P. J. (2019). The role of health literacy in diabetes knowledge, self-care, and glycemic control: A meta-analysis. *Journal of General Internal Medicine*, *34*(6), 1007–1017. https://doi.org/10.1007/s11606-019-04832-y

Morris, N. S., MacLean, C. D., & Littenberg, B. (2006). Literacy and health outcomes: A cross-sectional study in 1002 adults with diabetes. *BMC Family Practice*, *7*(49), 15.

Negarandeh, R., Mahmoodi, H., Noktehdan, H., Heshmat, R., & Shakibazadeh, E. (2013). Teach back and pictorial image educational strategies on knowledge about diabetes and medication/dietary adherence among low health literate patients with type 2 diabetes. *Primary Care Diabetes*, *7*(2), 111–1118. https://doi.org/10.1016/j.pcd.2012.11.001. PMID: 23195913

Okan, O., Bauer, U., Levin-Zamir, D., Pinheiro, P., & Sorensen, K. (2019). *International handbook of health literacy: Research, practice and policy across the life-span*. Policy Press.

Olesen, K. F., Reynheim, A. L., Joensen, L., Ridderstråle, M., Kayser, L., Maindal, H. T., Osborne, R. H., Skinner, T., & Willaing, I. (2017). Higher health literacy is associated with better glycemic control in adults with type 1 diabetes: A cohort study among 1399 Danes. *BMJ Open Diabetes Research & Care*, *5*(1), e000437. https://doi.org/10.1136/bmjdrc-2017-000437

Osborn, C., Paasche-Orlow, M., Bailey, S., & Wolf, M. (2011). The mechanisms linking health literacy to behavior and health status. *American Journal of Health Behavior*, *1*(35), 118–128.

Osborn, C. Y., Cavanaugh, K., Wallston, K. A., & Rothman, R. L. (2010). Self-efficacy links health literacy and numeracy to glycemic control. *Journal of Health Communication*, *15*(Suppl 2), 146–158. https://doi.org/10.1080/10810730.2010.499980

Paasche-Orlow, M. K., & Wolf, M. S. (2007). The causal pathways linking health literacy to health outcomes. *American Journal of Health Behaviour*, *31*, S19–S26.

Powers, M. A., Bardsley, J. K., Cypress, M., Funnell, M. M., Dixie Harms, D., Amy Hess-Fischl, A., Hooks, B., Isaacs, D., Mandel, E. D., Maryniuk, M. D., Norton, A., Rinker, J., Siminerio, L. M., & Uelmen, S. (2020, July). Diabetes self-management education and support in adults with type 2 diabetes: A consensus report of the American Diabetes Association, the Association of Diabetes Care & Education Specialists, the Academy of Nutrition and Dietetics, the American Academy. *Diabetes Care*, *43*(7), 1636−1649.

Schillinger, D., Grumbach, K., Piette, J., Wang, F., Osmond, D., Daher, C., Palacios, J., Sullivan, G. D., & Bindman, A. B. (2002). Association of health literacy with diabetes outcomes. *JAMA*, *288*(4), 475–482. https://doi.org/10.1001/jama.288.4.475

Sociedade Portuguesa de Diabetologia (SPD) – Diabetes: Factos e Números – O Ano de 2016, 2017 e 2018 − Relatório Anual do Observatório Nacional da Diabetes 12/2019.

Sorensen, K. (2019). Defining health literacy: Exploring differences and commonalities. In O. Okan, U. Bauer, D. Levin-Zamir, P. Pinheiro, & K. Sørensen (Eds.), *International handbook of health literacy: Research, practice and policy across the life-span* (pp. 5–20). Policy Press.

Sørensen, K., Pelikan, J. M., Röthlin, F., Ganahl, K., Slonska, Z., Doyle, G., Fullam, J., Kondilis, B., Agrafiotis, D., Uiters, E., Falcon, M., Mensing, M., Tchamov, K., van den Broucke, S., Brand, H., on behalf of the HLS-EU Consortium. (2015, December). Health literacy in Europe: Comparative results of the European health literacy survey (HLS-EU). *European Journal of Public Health*, *25*(6), 1053–1058. https://doi.org/10.1093/eurpub/ckv043

Sørensen, K., van den Broucke, S., Fullam, J., Doyle, G., Pelikan, J., Slonska, Z., & Brand, H. (2012). Health Literacy Project European health literacy and public health: A systematic review and integration of definitions and models. *BMC Public Health*, *80*(12), 80. https://doi.org/10.1186/1471-2458-12-80

Talevski, J., Wong Shee, A., Rasmussen, B., Kemp, G., & Beauchamp, A. (2020). Teach-back: A systematic review of implementation and impacts. *PLoS One*, *15*(4), e0231350. https://doi.org/10.1371/journal.pone.0231350

Toci, E., Burazeri, G., Jerliu, N., Sørensen, K., Ramadani, N., Hysa, B., & Brand, H. (2015). Health literacy, self-perceived health and self-reported chronic morbidity among older people in Kosovo. *Health Promotion International*, *30*(3), 667–674. https://doi.org/10.1093/heapro/dau009

World Health Organization (WHO). (1998). *Health Promotion Glossary*. WHO. https://www.who.int/healthpromotion/about/HPG/en/

Chapter 7

Digital Health Literacy and Young People: A Network of Mutual Influences

Cristina Vaz de Almeida[a], Diogo Franco Santos[b] and Patrícia Martins[c]

[a]*ISCSP – CAPP, President of Portuguese Health Literacy Society, Lisbon, Portugal*
[b]*Lapa Family Doctor UCSP – ACES Lisboa Central, Lisbon, Portugal*
[c]*Master and Specialist in Community Nursing at ARSLVT, Arnaldo Sampaio Public Health Unit of ACES Arco Ribeirinho, Lavradio, Portugal*

Abstract

Today's young people were born and raised in a digitally dominated world, therefore they quickly and intuitively navigate the web, which brings them undeniable advantages in the search for health information, but at the same time posing some risks. The authors conducted a narrative review of Portuguese and international scientific publications using the MeSH terms [Health literacy], [digital], [young people], [education] and [social media]. Among the various solutions presented, and considering the ease and speed to which young people are accustomed to when accessing digital information, the paths to be taken towards safe and effective navigation are related to solutions that promote a greater health literacy (HL). To bet on the promotion of HL in the younger generations is to invest in the improvement of their health and well-being, considering the **ACCESS** Young people are more likely to search and have access to health information through the digital environment, therefore it is important to reach them by means of interactive and appealing online content (e.g. short videos); **COMPREHENSION**, it is essential to disseminate reliable information and to involve their close social networks, including parents/legal guardians, social workers, teachers, among other community members; **USE** ensuring a correct and responsible use of health resources requires involving young people in the process of creating HL programs since its

Technology-Enhanced Healthcare Education:
Transformative Learning for Patient-Centric Health, 83–92
Copyright © 2024 by Cristina Vaz de Almeida, Diogo Franco Santos and Patricia Martins
Published under exclusive licence by Emerald Publishing Limited
doi:10.1108/978-1-83753-598-920231007

early steps. Results show that the digital promotion of HL as a valuable ·
tool to reach younger generations, who are avid consumers of social media
and many other online platforms.

Keywords: Young people; health literacy; digital health; education;
social media; digital information

Background

The World Health Organization (WHO) defines 'Health Literacy' (HL) as the
set of cognitive and social skills and one's ability to access, understand, assess
and use health information in order to promote and maintain good health.
Knowledge, motivation and personal skills are essential to a good understanding
of that information (WHO, 2013). To promote HL among young people is to
invest in the health and well-being of future generations. After all, today's young
people will be tomorrow's caregivers (Vaz de Almeida, 2022). Youth population is
defined by the WHO as those individuals aged between 10 and 24 years old, with
'teenagers' being aged 10–19 years old, and 'young people' aged 15–24 years old.
This is the stage of life in which behaviours and attitudes are strengthened, with
a likely impact on their future health (Silva et al., 2018).

Digital HL refers to one's ability to search, explore, understand and critically
assess health information from electronic resources, and apply this knowledge to solve a specific health problem (Direção-Geral da Saúde (DGS), 2019;
Norman & Skinner, 2006). Today's young people were born and grew up in a
digitally dominated world, and therefore can quickly and intuitively navigate
the internet. However, the lack of 'filters' regarding the suitability and relevance
of online information leads to a growing risk of misinformation and fake news.
Stellefson et al. (2011) emphasize, however, that today's broad access to online
health information does not necessarily correlate with better knowledge and assessment of such information. In other words, there is a growing concern for low digital
HL among young people, making it harder for them to better their health (Vaz de
Almeida, 2022; Sociedade Portuguesa de Literacia em Saúde & Miligrama –
Comunicação em Saúde; WHO, 2022). As an example, a study conducted in 2021
in Portugal (National School of Public Health – NOVA University Lisbon)
revealed that 44% of Portuguese university students have an inadequate or problematic level of HL, which is probably related to their socioeconomic background.
This study sheds light on the fact that, although current younger generations are
the most educated ever, their HL levels are still far from ideal (Pedro, 2022).

The global use of online social networks by young people reinforces the importance of reflecting on strategies to better their HL by the use of appealing and
dynamic ways through digital media.

Methods

The authors conducted a narrative review of Portuguese and international scientific publications using the MeSH terms [Health literacy], [digital], [young people],

[education] and [social media]. Inclusion criteria were related to their relevance to the subject of the article, which resulted in an extensive search, in contrast to a systematic review (Bryman, 2012). Priority was given to articles published in the last decade, although some older ones were also included given their relevance.

Discussion

HL Meets Education

Ghaddar et al. (2012) concluded that not only HL was positively associated with self-efficacy and online health information search (among high school students in South Texas) but also being exposed to credible online resources of health information contributed to higher levels of HL, which led them to suggest the incorporation of such resources into school curricula. Indeed, HL promotion through the access, understanding and use of health information seems to be of the utmost importance in adolescence, given that this is the stage of life in which health-promoting habits and behaviours are usually shaped, leading to better-informed decisions regarding their health and that of their peers, with a smarter use of the healthcare system and a consequent reduction in less favourable health outcomes. What's more, the few studies analyzing teenage literacy and HL have shown that low levels of literacy and HL are associated with risk behaviours, such as tobacco use, obesity or deviant behaviour.

Such conclusions are also supported by the above-mentioned Portuguese study (National School of Public Health, NOVA University Lisbon), which states that it is imperative to create health-promoting systems through HL programs targeting young people. In this sense, education and teaching institutions are privileged places for the implementation of such programs. Some large-scale projects have already been implemented at Portuguese schools, such as the National School Health Program (Direção-Geral da Saúde (DGS), 2005) and the Network of Health Promoting Schools. Other small-scale but equally important projects have also been developed in Portugal, such as the PEN (Period Empowerment Network) (Atlântica – Instituto Universitário, 2022a), to demystify issues related to menstruation, and the YHL (Youth Health Literacy) (Atlântica – Instituto Universitário, 2022b) focused on creating good practice guides for youth organizations.

The OECD (2017) report on 'The Future of Education and Skills 2030' named HL a core competency for the twenty-first century and a critical goal for education to empower citizens by increasing control over their own health. The WHO European Observatory on Health Systems and Policies, in its synthesis paper on HL in the education sector, identified several co-benefits for the education sector linked to HL, namely increased academic performance, health-related outcomes, and cost-effectiveness (McDaid, 2016). HL in schools requires the allocation of teaching time, the development of learning materials and teaching methods, as well as digital media and virtual learning environments (Okan et al., 2020). According to Sørensen and Okan (2020), to achieve high-quality health education, HL should be included in initial teacher training and school curricula. In fact, many schools already address concepts related to HL skills and action areas in their curricula, rather than introducing HL as a new concept, which means that it is possible to integrate HL into these preexisting topics (Okan et al., 2020).

Vaz de Almeida (2022) states that it is equally important to incorporate HL strategies in both the curricula of health courses and also in those of all other scientific areas, given that all students could potentially benefit from this action.

Active Learning

Check out the European Network of Health Promoting Schools:

https://www.schoolsforhealth.org/

It is also important to mention that, prior to designing a HL program, a survey must be carried out in order to assess the social, economic and geographic context and needs of the target young population, thus bridging the barriers related to access, understanding and use of health information. The authors of this article spoke at a webinar hosted by the Portuguese Society for Health Literacy in May 2022 on 'Young People and Health Literacy: What Challenges?', in which they highlighted the 'need for the development of school programs, in partnership with health institutions, in order to promote HL skills'. They also mentioned the relevance of 'creating an environment conducive to safety and well-being, encompassing the entire school community as well as the groups to which young people belong' as a HL-promoting measure (Nunes, Almeida & Belim, 2020; Nunes & Vaz de Almeida, 2020).

Active Learning

Webinar 'Young People and Health Literacy: What Challenges?':

https://www.youtube.com/watch?v=OwgagU6-NmM&ab_channel=Socied adePortuguesadeLiteraciaemSa%C3%BAde

---

Participation of Young People in HL Programs

Children, teenagers and young adults must be encouraged to actively participate in all stages of the development of HL programs, from their planning to the assessment of their results. These actions will ultimately contribute to their social and emotional growth while involving the whole school community and society. An active participation and inclusion of young people in the construction of HL programs seem essential for their success, whether or not they are digital (see Table 7.1).

According to UNESCO (2022), young people are encouraged to take action in every stage of any project development – from conception to completion and follow-up – in their communities, with the support and expansion of youth-led initiatives, as well as on the political agenda, voicing their concerns and issues. To this end, UNESCO also encourages the creation of Youth Spaces, aiming to

Table 7.1.   Measures to Promote the Participation and Inclusion of Young People in HL Programs.

- Listening and considering their interests and motivations about health
- Exploring and understanding the content of social media
- Making use of audiovisual media popular among them (e.g. videos, *stories*, *reels*)
- Taking into account their generational characteristics, such as the concern for sustainability and environmental protection or the awareness of LGBTQIA+ rights
- Involving them in school strategies and policies leading to healthier lifestyles and a greater understanding of risk factors
- Promoting peer education
- Developing co-creation workshops
- Making use of forms of artistic expression as strategies for health promotion and disease prevention
- Considering the importance of teleconsulting and messaging systems as relevant auxiliary tools in the communication and dissemination of information
- Considering the creation of a subject such as 'Health' or 'Health Literacy' at an early education stage (e.g. primary school)

Source: Own elaboration.

empower young people, foster and support their actions, promote partnerships, and ensure that they are given recognition and visibility.

The Digital Age

Nowadays, technologies are changing the way we live and relate to one another, as well as the way we teach or learn. The Digital Education Action Plan (2021–2027), announced in 2020 by Ursula von der Leyen, aims at acquiring digital skills and competencies from an early age that are necessary to responsibly use and interact with digital media, digital information and digital communication technologies through educational interventions (Okan et al., 2020).

ySKILLS (Youth Skills) is a project that aims to assess the digital skills of European teenagers as well as their evolution overtime (van Laar et al., 2022). To this end, between 2021 and 2023, a group of young people from six countries (Germany, Estonia, Finland, Italy, Poland and Portugal) are answering questions about digital access and skills (van Laar et al., 2022). Researchers Ponte et al. (2022), who carried out a Portuguese adaptation of this study, gathered 1,017 answers from teenagers aged between 12 and 17 years old. As far as daily online activities are concerned, 89% of them communicated with friends, 81% listened to music, 64% played games, 24% searched for news, 22% looked for new friends, 21% searched for information on physical health and treatments, 18% searched for information on mental health, 41% accessed the internet to learn new things, and 33% to practice something they are learning. On a school day, the average amount of time spent on the internet was 4 hours, with 41% of teenagers reporting that they were unable to tell whether a piece of information was actually true, with

35% not knowing how to assess whether a website was trustworthy (Ponte et al., 2022). It is important to highlight the fact that the COVID-19 pandemic was responsible for a boost in the search of online health services, which have become very popular worldwide ever since, captivating young people due to their easy access and convenience.

Active Learning

See here the 2021 results from the ySKILLS 2021 questionnaire reports: https://yskills.eu/publications/

Health information is made available and accessible in an almost unlimited way thanks to several digital communication platforms, spreading quickly through the internet and digital communication channels (Okan et al., 2020) and encouraging young people to adopt (digital) HL skills, such as social media literacy. Only in this way can they safely and appropriately surf the web in search of reliable health information (Bittlingmayer et al., 2020). In fact, as stated by the OECD (2017), current healthcare quality relies greatly on the ability to choose the most relevant information.

Dadaczynski et al. (2021) identified the sources of research used by students during the COVID-19 pandemic, having concluded that female students preferred social media and health websites, while male students mainly resorted to Wikipedia and other web-based encyclopedias, as well as YouTube. The use of social media was associated with a low critical ability to evaluate information, unlike what was seen with the use of public websites. Among other conclusions, Dadaczynski et al. emphasized the fact that, although university students seem to have good digital HL skills, many of them still struggle when assessing the credibility of online health information. Therefore, it is essential to empower them by means of personalized interventions, notwithstanding a need to improve the quality of that same information.

The previously mentioned study by Stellefson et al. (2011) concluded that some students showed reluctance to use interactive online applications in order to communicate with healthcare professionals. To be more precise, students did not mind searching the web for personal health information, however, they were somehow resistant to receiving individual feedback about personal health concerns or problems via interaction with a qualified medical professional. This issue may mirror web security issues affecting confidentiality and concern over data privacy, stressing the importance of understanding which health information sources cause them to feel uneasy. In this sense, early identification of young people's barriers, concerns and beliefs should be the first step in the development of HL-based interventions directed at them. Given the fact that younger generations (namely Generation Z and Alpha) are digital natives, they frequently experience the world through the screen of an electronic device, which makes it important to adopt appropriate and dynamic communication strategies within social media and other popular online platforms, so as to improve their access to health information.

Not surprisingly, teenagers do not seem to navigate the 'online health system' as thoroughly as adults do, since they are generally healthy and, therefore, do not worry about searching for health information as much (Ghaddar et al., 2012). Identifying the main challenges of young people's engagement with health information requires a critical reflection on how to make them better-informed citizens (SHE, 2014–2022). In order to do so, their profiles of action, life choices, trends, beliefs and concerns must necessarily be taken into account. What is more, not only do they currently have access to a wide range of information, but they are also frequently exposed to fake news, which constitutes an obstacle to HL (Vaz de Almeida, 2022) (see Table 7.2).

Working to improve HL among young people relies greatly on communication as a key element, as is true of most (if not all) areas of interest. A research study conducted within the scope of the Postgraduate Program 'Health Literacy in Practice' (ISPA, Lisbon) (Bernardes et al., 2021), analyzed a group of Millennials (Generation Y) from Portugal and Brazil with regard to their knowledge about hypertension, and it showed that they would rather receive information about this chronic disease by means of short 1-minute videos, rather than by any other formats (journals, magazines, e-books, email). Nowadays, these videos are mostly seen on social media, such as Instagram or TikTok, which are heavily used by children and teenagers, highlighting the need for regular audits in order to screen for fake news and harmful content. This matter also reinforces the need for appropriate parental digital skills, namely as supervisors of the online content their children are exposed to. Several online challenges that went viral worldwide, such as the 'Blue Whale Challenge', 'Momo', 'Goofy Man', 'Frozen Honey', 'Magnet' or the 'Blackout Challenge', posed several risks to those that participated in them. The latter started on TikTok and was heavily debated by the media as it resulted in the death of a 12-year-old British boy, Archie Battersbee (Sky, 2022). These challenges may have a negative impact on individual and

Table 7.2. Strategies for Fostering Young People's Interest in HL.

- Knowing how to listen to their needs, concerns and beliefs
- Helping with the management of their emotions, which are constantly changing (especially in the adolescent stage of life)
- Showing them that the digital world can be user-friendly when it comes to accessing health information
- Giving visibility to what they do and positively reinforce their character and ideas
- Giving feedback and commenting on their ideas, with appropriate and careful guidance
- Taking into account the characteristics of each young generation (X, Z and Alpha), with regard to their interests, motivations and concerns

Source: Vaz de Almeida (2022).

community health, and are a reminder of the importance of training parents and legal guardians in the acquisition of digital HL skills, in addition to monitoring their children's online activity.

Watzlawick et al. (2000) pointed out that 'everything is communication', and indeed it can come in several forms: physical, digital, verbal and non-verbal. It must be recalled that HL can be promoted not only by healthcare professionals working in clinics and hospitals but also at the institutional level and in health organizations, as well as in other contexts outside the scope of the health environment. As an example, the presence and representation of healthcare professionals in streaming platforms such as Netflix or HBO can also be a vehicle to disseminate trustworthy information, as a complement to other more 'conventional' ways, such as medical appointments, physical formats (e.g. books, magazines and newspapers) or information leaflets.

Active Learning

Learn more about cybersecurity at: https://www.seguranet.pt/

Conclusion

The association of higher levels of HL with better health outcomes has been clearly demonstrated in a great number of studies. The digital promotion of HL is a valuable tool to reach younger generations, who are avid consumers of social media and many other online platforms. The creation of multidisciplinary and intersectoral technical-scientific teams dedicated to the creation and promotion of HL programs involving all teaching and health institutions, social networks and the involving community – with specific training in models, strategies and techniques of HL – is an absolute necessity. Young people must be encouraged to participate in all steps of this process and have their perspectives listened to, in order to elaborate public policies that better reflect their real needs. Peer training is also a desirable goal since the success of HL programs is largely dependent on the capacity to plan, monitor and critically assess their progress and results. It is of the utmost importance to ensure that all young people, regardless of their social, economic, educational or geographical background, can benefit from such interventions. This way, empowered individuals will likely have a positive impact on the health of their peers and, on a larger scale, the community they live in. The global reach of digital media and its increasing use by young people worldwide make it the vehicle of choice to disseminate good health practices to forthcoming generations.

References

Atlântica – Instituto Universitário. (2022a). *Period Empowerment Network [PEN]*. https://www.uatlantica.pt/pen/

Atlântica – Instituto Universitário. (2022b). *Youth Health Literacy [YHL]*. https://www.uatlantica.pt/youth-health-literacy-yhl/

Bernardes, C. P., Santos, D. F., Taborda, P., & Barrambana, S. P. (2021). Literacia em Saúde na Prevenção da Hipertensão Arterial em Jovens Adultos. In *II Encontro de Literacia em Saúde na Prática*, 27 de novembro de 2021 (ISPA – Instituto Universitário). Video of the presentation (2:44:01 to 3:08:17): https://www.facebook.com/watch/live/?ref=watch_permalink&v=780340506697697

Bittlingmayer, U. H., Dadaczynski, K., Sahrai, D., van den Broucke, S., & Okan, O. (2020). Digitale Gesundheitskompetenz – Konzeptionelle Verortung, Erfassung und Förderung mit Fokus auf Kinder und Jugendliche. *Bundesgesundheitsbla, 63*, 176–184. https://doi.org/10.1007/s00103-019-03087-6

Bryman, A. (2012). *Social research methods* (4th ed.). Oxford University Press.

Dadaczynski, K., Okan, O., Messer, M., Leung, A. Y. M., Rosario, R., Darlington, E., & Rathmann, K. (2021). Digital health literacy and web-based information-seeking behaviors of university students in Germany during the COVID-19 pandemic: Cross-sectional Survey Study. *Journal of Medical Internet Research, 23*(1), e24097. https://doi.org/10.2196/24097

Direção-Geral da Saúde (DGS). (2005). *Programa Nacional de Saúde Escolar 2015*. DGS. https://observatorio-lisboa.eapn.pt/ficheiro/Programa-Nacional-de-Sa%C3%BAde-Escolar-2015.pdf

Direção-Geral da Saúde (DGS). (2019). *Manual de Boas Práticas, Literacia em Saúde – Capacitação dos Profissionais de Saúde*. https://www.dgs.pt/documentos-e-publicacoes/manual-de-boas-praticas-literacia-em-saude-capacitacao-dos-profissionais-de-saude-pdf.aspx

Direção-Geral da Saúde (DGS). (2020). *SeguraNet – Navegar em Segurança*. https://www.seguranet.pt/

Ghaddar, S. F., Valerio, M. A., Garcia, C. M., & Hansen, L. (2012). Adolescent health literacy: The importance of credible sources for online health information. *Journal of School Health, 82*(1), 28–36.

McDaid, D. (2016). *Investing in health literacy. What do we know about the co-benefits to the education sector of actions targeted at children and young people?* Policy Brief 19. World Health Organization Regional Office for Europe, European Observatory on Health Systems and Policies, Copenhagen.

Norman, C. D., & Skinner, H. A. (2006). eHealth literacy: Essential skills for consumer health in a networked world. *Journal of Medical Internet Research, 8*(2), e9.

Nunes, C., Almeida, C., & Belim, C. (2020). Health literacy in younger age groups: Health care perceptions: Informed people will be more prepared people. *Open Access Library Journal, 7*(3), 1–14. https://doi.org/10.4236/oalib.1106187; https://www.scirp.org/journal/paperinformation.aspx?paperid=98997h

Nunes, C., & Vaz de Almeida, C. (2020, October 30). Literacia em saúde em faixas etárias mais jovens: Perceções sobre cuidados com a saúde –Pessoas informadas serão pessoas mais preparadas. In *XIV Jornadas APDIS* (p. 42). Presentation selected for a Lucília Paiva Award. https://apdis.pt/publicacoes/index.php/jornadas/article/view/292/410

OECD. (2017). *Caring for quality in health. Lessons learnt from 15 reviews of health care quality*. OECD.

Okan, O., Bollweg, T. M., Berens, E.-M., Hurrelmann, K., Bauer, U., & Schaeffer, D. (2020). Coronavirus-related health literacy: A cross-sectional study in adults during the COVID-19 infodemic in Germany. *International Journal of Environmental Research and Public Health, 17*, 5503. https://doi.org/10.3390/ijerph17155503

Okan, O., Paakkari, L., & Dadaczynski, K. (2020). *Literacia em saúde nas escolas: Estado da arte*. SHE Factsheet 6. Schools for Health in Europe Network Foundation (SHE).

Pedro, A. R. (2022). Study: Health literacy in higher education: Challenges in Portugal. *APPSP, 18*, 2. http://appsp.org/site/assets/files/1231/newsletter_18.pdf

Ponte, C., Batista, S., & Baptista, R. (2022). *Results of the 1st series of the ySKILLS questionnaire (2021) – Portugal*. ySKILLS. https://www.fcsh.unl.pt/static/documentos/informacao/ySkills_Relatório_Portugal.pdf

SHE. (2014–2022). *Schools for health in Europe.* https://www.schoolsforhealth.org/

Silva, C. F., Rocha, P., & Santos, P. (2018). Consumption of licit and illicit substances in Portuguese young people: A population-based cross-sectional study. *Journal of International Medical Research*, *46*(8), 3042–3052. https://doi.org/10.1177/030006 0518767588

Sky, B. (2022, August 3). Archie, 12, tinha a morte marcada para as 11h00: O que todas as mães devem saber sobre ele e o TikTok. *CNN Portugal.* https://cnnportugal.iol.pt/archie-battersbee/tik-tok/archie-12-anos-tinha-a-morte-marcada-para-as-11h00-o-que-todas-as-maes-e-os-pais-do-mundo-devem-saber-sobre-ele-e-o-tiktok/20220803/62ea3ec50cf2 ea367d4832ca

Sociedade Portuguesa de Literacia em Saúde & Miligrama – Comunicação em Saúde (2022). *Webinar | Os Jovens e a Literacia em Saúde: Que Desafios?* https://www.youtube.com/watch?v=OwgagU6-NmM&t=1s&ab_channel=SociedadePortuguesadeL iteraciaemSa%C3%BAde

Sørensen, K., & Okan, O. (2020). *Health literacy. Health literacy of children and adolescents in school settings.* Global Health Literacy Acad./Fac. of Educational Science, Univ. Bielefeld/Internat. School Health Network.

Stellefson, M., Hanik, B., Chaney, B., Channey, D., Tennant, B., & Chvarria, E.A. (2011). eHealth literacy among college students: A systematic review with implications for eHealth education. *Journal of Medical Internet Research*, *13*(4), e10.

UNESCO. (2022). *Youth.* https://www.unesco.org/en/youth

van Laar, E., van Deursen, A. J. A. M., Helsper, E. J., & Schneider, L. S. (2022). *The youth digital skills performance tests: Report on the development of real-life tasks encompassing information navigation and processing, communication and interaction, and content creation and production skills.* ySKILLS.

Vaz de Almeida, C. (2022). *A literacia em saúde e os jovens.* PonteEditora. https://www.splsportugal.pt/_files/ugd/b5314a_dc2df8f771cd45f396e45b961bdab1f6.pdf

Watzlawick, P., Beavin, J. H., & Kackson, D. D. (2000). *Pragmatics of human communication* (11th ed.). Cultrix.

WHO. (2013). *Health literacy: The solid facts.* WHO.

WHO. (2022). *Recognize adolescence.* https://apps.who.int/adolescent/second-decade/section2/page1/recognizing-adolescence.htm

Chapter 8

WalkingPad: The Patient Experience in Peripheral Artery Disease

Ivone Fernandes Santos Silva

*Instituto de Ciência Abel Salazar, Porto, Portugal; Cardiovascular Research Group –
UMIB, Porto, Portugal*

Abstract

Peripheral arterial disease (PAD) is an occlusive atherosclerotic disease
that affects blood vessels and reduces blood flow in the lower limbs. It is
estimated that around 200 million people worldwide suffered from it, with
a significant number of older people affected. Walking is one of the first-
line therapeutic measures for intermittent claudication (IC) in patients with
PAD. Supervised Exercise Therapy (SET) programs effectively increase
walking distances, however, remain an underutilized tool because they
are not readily available in most clinical centres, are extremely expensive,
and patient participation is low mainly due to socioeconomic constraints.
Home-based Exercise Therapy (HBET) programs are an effective and low-
cost alternative to improve both the functional capacity and quality of life
(QoL) of patients with IC, as they are performed in the patient's area of
residence and not in the hospital. The WalkingPad program conciliated
a smartphone app – the WalkingPad app – with behaviour change intervention to increase walking distances and decrease walking impairment as
well to improve QoL at 6 months.

Keywords: Peripheral arterial disease; intermittent claudication; exercise;
home-based; M-Health

Technology-Enhanced Healthcare Education:
Transformative Learning for Patient-Centric Health, 93–114
Copyright © 2024 by Ivone Fernandes Santos Silva
Published under exclusive licence by Emerald Publishing Limited
doi:10.1108/978-1-83753-598-920231008

Introduction

PAD is a cardiovascular disorder that affects more than 200 million people worldwide. It is associated with the occlusion of peripheral arteries and predominantly affects the arteries of the lower limbs (G. Santulli, 2008). PAD causes symptoms such as IC, reducing patients' functional capacity due to pain that is induced by muscle ischemia during exercise (walking) and is relieved at rest. This condition is also associated with increased cardiovascular morbidity and mortality due to the ongoing generalized atherosclerotic process (W. Teijink, 2018).

Improving functional capacity, QoL, reducing symptoms, morbidity, and mortality are the main focuses of PAD management. Modification of risk factors and exercise therapy are first-line therapy in all guidelines (M. D. Gerhard-Herman et al., 2016).

Exercise therapy programs have been strongly recommended for patients with PAD and IC because they increase pain-free walking distance and enhance QoL. Current PAD guidelines recommend that exercise training, in the form of walking, should be performed for a minimum of 30–45 minutes per session, 3–4 times per week, for a period not less than 12 weeks (M. D. Gerhard-Herman et al., 2016)

SET has been the gold standard, it takes place in a hospital or outpatient setting, where intermittent walking exercise is used as a treatment modality and is directly supervised by qualified health professionals (Gerhard-Herman et al., 2017; Norgren et al., 2007). However, due to several limitations associated with the access, time available, distances, and costs involved for patients as well as the availability of SET in clinical centres, HBET has emerged as a structured, unsupervised, and self-directed option that takes place in the personal environment of the patient and not in a clinical setting (Gerhard-Herman et al., 2017).

HBET programs may provide an effective alternative when SET programs are not available. These are structured programs that may include a monitoring component (e.g. logbooks or electronic monitoring devices) and personalized walking advice.

The rate of adherence to exercise therapy programs is low mainly due to patients' lack of motivation, but also because of difficulties associated with health status and lack of results (Chetter, 2016; A. Harzand et al., 2020).

However, in Golledge et al. (2019) meta-analysis, HBET programs that included a motivational intervention significantly improved walking performance and physical activity in patients with PAD (J. Golledge et al., 2019).

Thus, it is imperative that we develop strategies to improve motivation and adherence to physical exercise in this population. M-Health technologies offer valuable tools that can be used for monitoring patients in HBET programs. Geographical information systems (GIS) (such as Google Maps) are home-based, inexpensive, and easy to use applications which are accessible to a wide range of the population. In a study by M. M. McDermott et al. (2018), Google Maps provided enough accuracy for monitoring PAD home-based exercise, delivering a landmarks-based method that objectively measured patients and; adherence to an exercise plan.

In addition, the use of M-health tools for self-monitoring can be a way to motivate patients and drive initial behaviour change.

Studies describing the use of M-Health in PAD, in particular the use of mobile applications, are very limited (J. W. Hinnen, 2021). To date, only two apps were developed for this purpose (CReTe, Spain, 2014 and JBZetje, the Netherlands, 2021). Both collect data from exercise sessions, such as walking distance, the number of stops, reasons for stopping, time spent walking, and speed. They also allow patients to access their walking history and progression. In an effort to fill the gaps found in these applications, we developed a mobile application to assist patients with PAD while performing exercise therapy.

We have developed the WalkingPad program that includes – The WalkingPad app. We believe that HBET programs for PAD patients, supported by an M-Health tool that uses behaviour change strategies, such as self-monitoring, feedback, and goal setting, may be effective in promoting exercise therapy. Our program records patients walking history and provides progression feedback and self-monitoring and has the ability to customize routes according to patients' preference and location.

What Do Patients Need to Adhere to an Exercise Prescription?

Customization, specification, and detail: A qualitative study found that patients report a lack of understanding of the effectiveness of walking, desire personalized walking guidelines, and complain of a lack of specific walking instructions (e.g. Should I continue to walk when the pain appears? Should I strain?) (Galea et al., 2013). In addition, patients still have uncertainties about the disease and doubts about the treatment (Striberger et al., 2020) that can contribute to non-adherence to physical exercise. Therefore, first, the exercise prescription must be personalized and include specific guidelines as if it were a drug prescription.

Motives for walking are more than just improving health: When we prescribe exercise we are asking patients to seek pain and not avoid it. This principle is contrary to the human nature of seeking pleasure and avoiding pain (Ekkekakis & Dafermos, 2012). Thus, motivating people with PAD and IC to practice physical exercise is a challenge since, as they feel pain when walking, it is natural for them to avoid doing so. Thus, health professionals must help patients find motives and reasons to walk, in addition to improving health and ameliorating PAD symptoms, because this concept is difficult to 'see', quantify, and objectify. The goal needs to be more objective, concrete, and adapted to the patients' goals and life priorities (e.g. being able to play with grandchildren). Motives are the drivers of volitional behaviour as they help to set priorities and allocate resources for behaviour change. To engage in behaviour that you know in advance will cause pain, and you won't get immediate satisfaction or pleasure, motives must get as close as possible to the intrinsic goals people value. On the other hand, the reasons for maintaining a behaviour are often different from the reasons that lead people to make the initial changes. Thus, the behaviour will be more easily integrated, and the likelihood of long-term adherence will be greater if it meets the goals, values, and meanings of the person's life, and if it allows regular gratification for its practice and not just the experience of change (Kwasnicka et al., 2016).

Prescribing pleasure, satisfaction, positive emotions, self-care, and self-love and not just physical exercise: The exercise prescription should include the suggestion of pleasure and positive emotions that will arise during exercise (Segar & Richardson, 2014). Hence, framing walking as a strategy to improve well-being and pleasure explicitly encourages people to determine how they want to walk (e.g. influences their intensity) (Segar & Richardson, 2014). Thus, when people are asked to self-regulate their walking pace based on maintaining positive feelings, they select intensities that approach the ventilatory threshold (Rose & Parfitt, 2008). Therefore, health professionals need not worry about people choosing to walk slowly to maintain well-being and positive emotions.

These aforementioned strategies help people to 'look' at exercise differently, to give it another meaning and value (Henderson et al., 2013; Segar et al., 2011). This reframing is fundamental to the self-regulation of sustainability because, by pursuing autonomous goals that reflect the most important and valuable parts of people's lives, people optimize the ongoing behavioural pursuit (Gaudreau et al., 2012). Thus, this approach promotes autonomous motivation, which is a type of motivation most strongly associated with the sustainability of regular walking (Teixeira et al., 2012). In turn, prescribing medically based 'doses' of physical activity to optimize health outcomes undermines adherence by inadvertently thwarting autonomy and positive affect and increasing negative affect, which leads to exercise avoidance and non-adherence (Ekkekakis, 2013).

The objective of WalkingPad was to find what makes an HBET prescription easier to comply with: What do patients want and need to adhere easily to an exercise prescription? We worked on a development and evaluation of a mobile application – the WalkingPad app – aimed at promoting adherence to physical exercise among patients with PAD (Silva et al., 2022).

Materials and Methods

This is a single-center, prospective, two-arm, single-blinded (to patients) randomized controlled trial (RCT) reported in line with the CONSORT checklist (Schulz et al., 2010). This study was approved by the Research Ethics Committee of the hospital where the study was conducted on 22 October 2019 (reference: 069-DEFI/068-CES). Each patient was informed of the risks and benefits involved in the study and signed written informed consent for participation. The RCT protocol was registered on the U.S. National Library of Medicine (ClinicalTrials.gov) with the identifier NCT04749732 on 10 February 2021.

Participant Recruitment and Eligibility

Participants were identified between January and March 2021, by consulting the medical records of patients enrolled in the Angiology and Vascular Surgery consultation. Patients aged between 50 and 80 years and with MWD between 50 and 500 metres were selected. Eligibility for the study was tested by consulting medical records and by a screening assessment (time 0) (in the case of objective criteria such as walking distance). The inclusion criteria were the following: (1) PAD with IC (Fontaine II or Rutherford 1–3) due to atherosclerotic disease; (2) Ankle Brachial Index (ABI) below 0.9 at rest or below 0.73 after exercise (20% decrease); (3) age range between 50 and 80 years; and (4) MWD in treadmill test between 50 and 500 metres. Exclusion criteria were the following: (1) asymptomatic PAD; (2) critical ischemia (Fontaine III/IV or Rutherford 4–6); (3) previous lower extremity vascular surgery, angioplasty, or lumbar sympathectomy; (4) any condition other than PAD that limits walking; (5) unstable angina or myocardial infarction diagnosed in the last 6 months; (6) inability to obtain ABI measure due to non-compressible vessels; (7) use of cilostazol and pentoxifylline initiated within 3 months before the investigation; (8) active cancer, renal disease, or liver disease; (9) severe chronic obstructive pulmonary disease (GOLD stage III/IV); (10) severe congestive heart failure (NYHA class III/IV); (11) diagnosis of a psychiatric disease that impairs daily life activities and/or with medical records of decompensation episodes in the last year and/or non-adherence to drug therapy; (12) cognitive impairment (Mini-Mental State Examination (MMSE) ≤15 for illiterate patients, 22 for those with 1–11 years of schooling; 27 for >11 years). For those who accepted participation in the study, a screening assessment (time 0 – before allocation) to determine particular and specific eligibility criteria, was scheduled at the hospital where a clinical, physical, and hemodynamic assessment, as well as a screening measure of cognitive function, were applied.

Then, randomization was carried out in blocks with four strata, and the eligible participants were randomly assigned to two groups, in blocks of multiples of five, and stratified according to (i) age (50–65 years old; 66–80 years old); and (ii) MWD at baseline (time 0) (50–275 metres; 276–500 metres). Participants were unaware of the group to which they were assigned: control group (CG) or experimental group (EG). After allocation, participants were evaluated with psychological measures and received a physical exercise prescription to be performed in their area of residence and a brief face-to-face behavioural change and motivational intervention. The study lasted 6 months/24 weeks and involved four hospital visits: time 0 (baseline – to verify objective inclusion and exclusion criteria), time 1 (2 weeks after time 0: baseline), time 2 (3 months after time 1), and time 3 (6 months after time 1). Fig. 8.1 shows the study flowchart.

Interventions

All participants were undergoing standard treatment for PAD and IC, according to the guidelines of the American College of Cardiology/American Heart Association Task Force on Clinical Practice Guidelines (AHA/ACC) (Aboyans et al., 2018; Gerhard-Herman et al., 2016; Norgren et al., 2007; Treat-Jacobson et al., 2019). Participants received a personalized physical exercise prescription to be

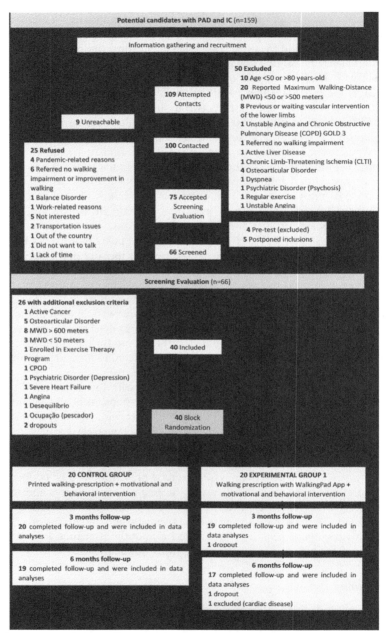

Fig. 8.1.   Potential Candidates With PAD and IC (*n* = 159).

performed in their area of residence for 6 months and a behavioural and motivational change intervention – the WalkingPad intervention. The physical exercise prescription consists of walking exercise, with a duration greater than 30 minutes per session and a frequency of at least three sessions per week. Near-maximal pain during training was the claudication pain endpoint. The brief face-to-face behavioural change intervention included an education component about PAD and a behavioural intervention based on Self Determination Theory and motivational interview principles. Patients received two face-to-face sessions (at time 1 and time 2) conducted by a health psychologist, for a total of four hours (2:00 each session). In addition, booster phone calls were provided to promote long-term adherence to the physical exercise prescription.

Control Group

Participants assigned to this group received a self-fulfilling walking practice diary to monitor and record walking sessions. The diary has the following indicators: frequency (date) and duration of the walking session, the number of stops and the level of well-being (ranging between 0 very bad and 10 very good) to be filled in each walking session.

Experimental Group

Participants assigned to this group received a smartphone (Samsung Galaxy A41 SM-A415F/DSN, Vietnam) with a WalkingPad app (smartphone application). In addition to providing access to the patients' walking history and progression (e.g. walking frequency, duration, number of stops, and velocity), allowing self-monitorization and tailored feedback, this app also permits the personalization of the walking route, according to the patient walking capacity, measured through a standardized test, and their preferred and familiarized location, promoting a greater adherence to the physical exercise. Details about the WalkingPad app will be described elsewhere. Along with the WalkingPad app, a web platform (WalkingPad web platform) was created allowing collaboration between different actors (health professionals, researchers, and engineers) in monitoring patient adherence, promoting patients' responsibility in their treatment strategy, and providing feedback during booster phone calls (Fig. 8.2).

Primary Outcomes Measures

The primary outcomes were between-group differences over 6 months in the WalkingPad program-induced change in PFWD, FWD, MWD, and 6MWD. PFWD is defined as the distance walked at the onset of claudication pain. The FWD is defined as the distance at which a patient prefers to stop because of claudication pain. The MWD is defined as the distance at which claudication pain becomes so severe that the patient is forced to stop. The 6MWD is defined as the distance the patient can walk in 6 minutes, regardless of stops.

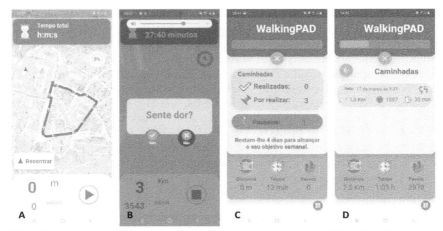

Fig. 8.2.   (A) Personalized Route; (B) Reason for Stopping "Do You Feel Pain?"; (C) and (D) Walking History and Progression.

The Treadmill Test (Kruidenier et al., 2009) was used with the modified Gardner-Skinner Treadmill Protocol, where participants begin to walk on the treadmill at 1 km/h with a 0% grade. After 2 minutes the speed is increased to 1.6 km/h, at 0% grade. Then the speed is increased by 0.8 km/h every 2 minutes until reaching 3.2 km/h. After reaching 3.2 km/h, the speed is kept constant, and the grade is increased by 2% every 2 minutes.

The 6-Minute Walk Test (6MWT) was performed to evaluate the functional capacity of the individual to walk over a total of 6 minutes on a 100-ft (≈30 m) hallway (Treat-Jacobson et al., 2019) according to the American Thoracic Society guidelines (Anderson et al., 2009).

Secondary Outcomes Measures

Vascular Disease-Specific Quality of Life Questionnaire (VAscuQoL-6) (Correia et al., 2018; Kumlien et al., 2017; Nordanstig et al., 2014) was used to assess health-related QoL in patients with PAD, consisting of six items with different response scales. The total score ranges from 6 to 24, with higher results corresponding to a higher QoL associated with vascular disease symptoms. Cronbach's alpha in this study was 0.70.

Walking Impairment Questionnaire (WIQ) (Nicolaï et al., 2009) was used to assess the daily walking ability of patients in three domains: distance (distances the patient can walk), speed (the speed the patient can walk), and climbing stairs (number of stairs that the patient can climb without stopping), in a 5-point Likert scale (none, slight, some, quite difficult, and unable). The distance comprises 7 items with a total score ranging from 0 to 28, with the highest results corresponding to a greater walked distance. Cronbach's alpha in this study was 0.84. Speed has 4 items with a total score ranging from 0 to 16, with higher values indicating greater speed; Cronbach's alpha in this study was 0.64. Climbing stairs contain three items with a total score ranging from 0 to 12, with higher results indicating a greater ability to climb stairs. Cronbach's alpha in this study was 0.88.

Sociodemographic and clinical data were collected from the participants' clinical medical records and through a clinical interview.

Cognitive function was measured through the MMSE (Kim et al., 1975) which includes tests of orientation, attention, memory, language, and visual-spatial skills. The total score ranges from 0 to 30, and higher results correspond to better cognitive function. It was applied at baseline (time 0) as part of the screening assessment to ascertain exclusion criteria.

Physical measures include the assessment of ABI (McDermott et al., 2001; Resnick et al., 2004) before and after the treadmill test by measuring the systolic pressures at the brachial artery, anterior tibial artery, and posterior tibial artery, in the supine position, in millimetres of mercury (mmHg), using a Doppler device.

Hand Grip Strength (HGS) is a basic measure for determining musculoskeletal function, as well as weakness and disability (Bohannon & Magasi, 2015). The HGS produces an isometric strength measure that allows the identification of the muscular weakness of the upper limb and provides an indication of the overall strength since it reflects the strength of the lower limbs.

Body composition: Weight, body mass index, body fat percentage, visceral fat level, skeletal muscle percentage, and resting metabolism were measured through a bioimpedance scale. Height was measured using a tape measure.

Statistical Analysis

Descriptive statistics were used to summarize sociodemographic and clinical variables and primary and secondary outcomes. Nominal/dichotomous/categorical data were presented in numbers and percentages and compared between the EG and the CG using the chi-square test (X^2). Continuous data were presented as mean and standard deviation and compared between groups using the Mann–Whitney U-test. A one-way repeated measure of variance (ANOVA) was conducted to test the interaction between groups (between-subjects factor) and between the three assessment points (in-subjects factor) for each primary and secondary outcome. Mauchly's sphericity test was used to verify the sphericity assumption (sphericity assumed if $p > 0.05$). If non-sphericity was present, and to combat violation of the sphericity assumption, the results were reported with Greenhouse-Geisser correction. If there were statistically significant effects over the three assessment moments, *post hoc* tests and Bonferroni tests adjusted to pairwise comparisons were performed to find out which evaluation moment at which the effect was significant. Change in primary and secondary outcomes were analyzed by calculating the difference between the three moments (Δ = t1 score – t3 score; Δ = t1 score – t2 score; Δ = t2 score – t3 score). Analyses were performed on an intention-to-treat basis. During the treadmill test, some patients showed no need to rest or stop after the onset of initial pain. Therefore, the number of participants is smaller in the variables PFWD and the FWD than in the variable MWD. Effect size measures and statistical power ($1 - \beta$) were presented. The following thresholds were considered for partial eta-squared (np^2): above 0.01 = small effect size, above 0.06 = medium effect size, above 0.14 = large effect size; and the following were adopted for Cohen's *d*: above 0.20 = small, above 0.50 = medium, and above 0.80 = large effect size. Statistical Package for Social Sciences (SPSS) version 25.0 (IBM SPSS Inc., Chicago, IL) was used to perform all analyses. *P*-values < 0.05 were considered statistically significant throughout.

Results

Sociodemographic and Clinical Characterization

From the clinical medical records consultation, 268 patients were identified, 119 were invited to attend a screening evaluation at the hospital to verify the presence of other inclusion criteria (time 0: at baseline) and only 73 were included in the study randomized and allocated to one of the two groups (Fig. 8.1). Of these, only 60 participated in the three assessment moments. Excluded patients differ significantly from included patients in the following variables: living status ($X^2(1) = 8.529$, $p = 0.003$), cilostazol intake ($X^2(1) = 5.294$, $p = 0.021$), smoking history ($X^2(1) = 4.416$, $p = 0.036$), time since quitting smoking ($t(53) = 2.087$, $p = 0.042$), chronic renal disease ($X^2(1) = 5.319$, $p = 0.021$), BMI ($t(113) = -6.653$, $p < 0.001$), body muscle ($t(113) = -2.321$, $p = 0.022$), metabolic basal rate ($t(113) = -2.292$, $p = 0.024$), initial pain score rate ($t(99) = 3.801$, $p < 0.001$), and final pain score rate ($t(103) = -2.294$, $p = 0.004$), in treadmill test, that is, the group of excluded patients has more patients living alone, who have quit smoking longer and with stronger initial pain in the treadmill test. The group of patients included has more patients using cilostazol, with a history of smoking, fewer patients with chronic kidney disease and less muscle mass, less initial pain but greater final pain, and higher BMI and basal metabolic rate.

Sample Characterization and Differences Between CG and EG Patients

There were found two differences in clinical characteristics between patients from the CG when compared with patients from the EG. The CG has more patients taking Clopidogrel ($X^2(1) = 5.192$, $p = 0.023$) than patients in the EG. In turn, CG has more patients taking Cilostazol ($X^2(1) = 5.455$, $p = 0.020$). Patients from the CG rated a higher level of functional pain during the treadmill test ($t(53) = 2.324$, $p = 0.024$) (Table 8.1).

Primary and Secondary Outcomes Characterization and Differences Between CG and EG Patients

There were no differences in primary and secondary outcomes between patients assigned to the CG or the EG, indicating that the groups were similar ($p = 0.05$) at baseline in each treadmill measure: MWD, PFWD, FWD, and the 6MWT, as well as walking impairments (distance, speed, and stairs climbing) and reported QoL.

Table 8.1. Sociodemographic and Clinical Variables Characterization and Differences Between Excluded and Included Patients.

Dichotomous Variables		Total Sample (*n* = 66)	Excluded Patients (*n* = 26)	Included Patients (*n* = 40)	Statistical Tests	
Sociodemographic		*n* (%)	*n* (%)	*n* (%)	X^2 (df)	*p*-value
Sex	Male	56 (84.8)	21 (80.0)	35 (87.5)	0.555 (1)	0.456
	Female	10 (15.2)	5 (19.2)	5 (12.5)		
Living status	Alone	8 (12.1)	7 (26.9)	1 (2.5)	8.824 (1)	**0.005**
	With others	58 (87.9)	19 (73.1)	39 (97.5)		
Professional profile	Active/ unemployed	24 (36.4)	10 (38.5)	14 (35.0)	0.082 (1)	0.799
	Retired	42 (63.6	16 (61.5)	26 (65.0)		
Marital status	Married	46 (69.7)	16 (61.5)	30 (75.0)	–	–
	Civil union	1 (1.5)	1 (3.8)	0 (0.0)	–	–
	Widowed	6 (9.1)	2 (7.7)	4 (10.0)	–	–
	Single	4 (6.1)	3 (11.5)	1 (2.5)	–	–
	Divorced	9 (13.6)	4 (15.4)	5 (12.5)	–	–
Marital status	With spouse	47 (71.2)	17 (65.3)	30 (75.0)	0.711 (1)	0.399
	Without spouse	19 (28.8)	9 (34.6)	10 (25.0)		
Children	Yes	5 (7.6)	3 (11.5)	2 (5.0)	0.962 (1)	0.327
	No	61 (92.4)	23 (88.5)	38 (95.0)		
Residency	Rural	11 (16.7)	5 (19.2)	6 (15.0)	0.203 (1)	0.652
	Urban	55 (83.3)	21 (80.8)	34 (85.0)		
Mobile phone	No	2 (3.7)	2 (14.3)	0 (0.0)	–	–
	Yes, smartphone	13 (24.1)	10 (71.4)	29 (72.5)	0.578 (1)	0.447
	Yes, older phone	39 (72.2)	2 (14.3)	11 (27.5)		
Clinical						
Hypertension	No	10 (15.2)	6 (23.1)	4 (10)	2.096 (1)	0.148
	Yes	56 (84.8)	20 (76.9)	36 (90.0)		
Colesterol	No	10 (15.2)	3 (11.5)	7 (17.5)	0.436 (1)	0.509
	Yes	56 (84.8)	23 (88.5)	33 (82.5)		

(*Continued*)

Table 8.1.   (*Continued*)

Dichotomous Variables		Total Sample (*n* = 66)	Excluded Patients (*n* = 26)	Included Patients (*n* = 40)	Statistical Tests
Obesity (BMI > 30)	No	44 (66.7)	20 (76.9)	24 (60.0)	2.031 (1) 0.154
	Yes	22 (33.3)	6 (23.1)	16 (40.0)	
Diabetes mellitus type 1	No	65 (98.5)	25 (96.2)	40 (100.0)	1.562 (1) 0.211
	Yes	1 (1.5)	1 (3.8)	0 (0.0)	
Diabetes mellitus type 2	No	34 (51.5)	15 (57.7)	19 (47.5)	0.655 (1) 0.418
	Yes	32 (48.5)	11 (42.3)	21 (52.5)	
Smoking history (active or former)	No	5 (7.6)	2 (7.7)	3 (7.5)	0.001 (1) 0.977
	Yes	61 (92.4)	24 (92.3)	37 (92.5)	
Cerebrovascular disease (Stroke, TIA)	No	56 (84.8)	21 (80.8)	35 (87.5)	0.555 (1) 0.456
	Yes	10 (15.2)	5 (19.2)	5 (12.5)	
Depression/ anxiety	No	61 (92.4)	23 (88.5)	38 (95.0)	0.962 (1) 0.327
	Yes	5 (7.6)	3 (11.5)	2 (5.0)	
Ischemic heart disease	No	51 (77.3)	20 (76.9)	31 (77.5)	0.003 (1) 0.956
	Yes	15 (22.7)	6 (23.1)	9 (22.5)	
COPD	No	50 (75.8)	20 (76.9)	30 (75.0)	0.032 (1) 0.858
	Yes	16 (24.2)	6 (23.1)	10 (25.0)	
Heart faillure	No	60 (90.9)	23 (88.5)	37 (92.5)	0.311 (1) 0.577
	Yes	6 (9.1)	3 (11.5)	3 (75.5)	
Chronic renal disease	No	62 (93.9)	23 (88.5)	39 (97.5)	2.261 (1) 0.133
	Yes	4 (6.1)	3 (11.5)	1 (2.5)	
Osteoarticular disease	No	52 (78.8)	19 (73.1)	33 (82.5)	0.837 (1) 0.360
	Yes	14 (21.2)	7 (26.9)	7 (17.5)	
Neurologic disease	No	65 (98.5)	25 (96.2)	40 (100.0)	1.562 (1) 0.211
	Yes	1 (1.5)	1 (3.8)	0 (0.0)	
Liver disease	No	59 (89.4)	22 (84.6)	37 (92.5)	1.033 (1) 0.309
	Yes	7 (10.6)	4 (15.4)	3 (7.5)	
Active cancer	No	65 (98.5)	25 (96.2)	40 (100.0)	1.562 (1) 0.211
	Yes	1 (1.5)	1 (3.8)	0 (0.0)	

Table 8.1. (*Continued*)

Dichotomous Variables		Total Sample (*n* = 66)	Excluded Patients (*n* = 26)	Included Patients (*n* = 40)	Statistical Tests	
Others	No	42 (63.6)	17 (65.4)	25 (62.5)		
	Yes	24 (36.4)	9 (34.6)	15 (37.5)		
Surgical history	No	19 (28.8)	9 (34.6)	10 (25.0)	0.711 (1)	0.399
	Yes	47 (71.2)	17 (65.4)	30 (75.0)		
Medication						
Acetylsalicylic acid	No	13 (19.7)	6 (23.1)	7 (17.5)	0.310 (1)	0.578
	Yes	53 (80.3)	20 (76.9)	33 (82.5)		
Clopidogrel	No	55 (83.3)	20 (76.9)	35 (87.5)	1.269 (1)	0.260
	Yes	11 (16.7)	6 (23.1)	5 (12.5)		
Statins	No	9 (13.6)	4 (15.4)	5 (12.5)	0.111 (1)	0.739
	Yes	57 (86.4)	22 (84.6)	35 (87.5)		
Pentoxifilin	No	53 (80.3)	20 (76.9)	33 (82.5)	0.310 (1)	0.578
	Yes	13 (19.7)	6 (23.1)	7 (17.5)		
Insulin	No	59 (89.4)	24 (92.3)	35 (87.5)	0.384 (1)	0.535
	Yes	7 (10.6)	2 (7.7)	5 (12.5)		
Cilostazol	No	54 (81.8)	25 (96.2)	29 (72.5)	5.927 (1)	**0.015**
	Yes	12 (18.2)	1 (3.8)	11 (27.5)		
NOACs	No	56 (84.8)	20 (76.9)	36 (90.0)	2.096 (1)	0.148
	Yes	10 (15.2)	6 (23.1)	4 (10.0)		
Warfarin	No	63 (95.5)	26 (100.0)	37 (92.5)	2.043 (1)	0.153
	Yes	3 (4.5)	0 (0.0)	3 (7.5)		
Oral antidiabetic agents	No	37 (56.1)	18 (69.2)	19 (47.5)	3.021 (1)	0.082
	Yes	29 (43.9)	8 (30.8)	21 (52.5)		
Beta-blockers	No	47 (71.2)	19 (73.1)	28 (70.0)	0.073 (1)	0.787
	Yes	19 (28.8)	7 (26.9)	12 (30.0)		
Antihipertensive agents	No	18 (27.3)	8 (30.8)	10 (25.0)	0.264 (1)	0.607
	Yes	48 (72.7)	18 (69.2)	30 (75.0)		
Others	No	30 (45.5)	11 (42.3)	19 (47.5)	0.171 (1)	0.679
	Yes	36 (54.5)	15 (57.7)	21 (52.5)		
New medication started in the last 3 months	No	59 (89.4)	22 (84.6)	37 (92.5)	1.033 (1)	0.309
	Yes	7 (10.6)	4 (15.4)	3 (7.5)		

(*Continued*)

Table 8.1.   (*Continued*)

Dichotomous Variables		Total Sample (*n* = 66)	Excluded Patients (*n* = 26)	Included Patients (*n* = 40)	Statistical Tests	
Lifestyle						
Drinking history	No	20 (30.3)	12 (46.2)	8 (20.0)	5.103 (1)	**0.09224**
	Yes	46 (69.7)	14 (53.8)	32 (80.0)		
Smoking history	Active smoker	27 (40.9)	9 (34.6)	18 (45.0)	0.026	0.873
	Former smoker	34 (51.5)	15 (57.7)	19 (47.5)		
	Never smoked	5 (7.6)	2 (7.7)	3 (7.5)		
Pain – Edimburg Questionnaire						
Pain or discomfort in your legs while you walk	No	0 (0.0)	0 (0.0)	0 (0.0)		
	Yes	100 (0.0)	100 (0.0)	100 (0.0)		
Pain when you are standing still or sitting	No	58 (87.9)	23 (88.5)	35 (87.5)	0.014 (1)	0.907
	Yes	8 (12.1)	3 (11.5)	5 (12.5)		
Pain if you walk uphill or hurry	No	11 (16.7)	8 (30.8)	3 (7.5)	6.143 (1)	**0.013**
	Yes	55 (83.3)	18 (69.2)	37 (92.5)		
Pain at an ordinary pace at the level	No	4 (6.1)	2 (7.7)	2 (5.0)	0.201 (1)	0.654
	Yes	62 (93.9)	24 (92.3)	38 (95.0)		
Pain continues for more than 10 minutes after you stop	No	6 (9.1)	5 (1)	1 (2.5)	5.337 (1)	**0.021**
	Yes	60 (90.9)	21 (80.8)	39 (97.5)		
Pain is more intense in … leg	Right	25 (37.9)	10 (38.5)	15 (37.5)		
	Left	31 (47.0)	12 (46.2)	19 (47.5)		
	Both	10 (15.2)	4 (15.4)	6 (15.0)		
IPAQ						
IPAQ categories	Insufficiently active	54 (81.8)	22 (84.6)	32 (80.0)		
	Moderately active	7 (10.6)	1 (3.8)	6 (15.0)		
	Vigorously active	5 (7.6)	3 (11.5)	2 (5.0)		

Table 8.1. (*Continued*)

Dichotomous Variables		Total Sample (*n* = 66)	Excluded Patients (*n* = 26)	Included Patients (*n* = 40)	Statistical Tests
IPAQ _two groups	Insufficiently active	53 (80.3)	22 (84.6)	31 (77.5)	0.504 (1) 0.478
	Moderate/ vigorously active	13 (19.7)	4 (15.4)	9 (22.5)	
BMI					
BMI categories	Normal weight	19 (28.8)	7 (26.9)	12 (30.0)	
	Pre-obesity	26 (39.4)	13 (50.0)	13 (32.5)	
	Obesity class 1	18 (27.3)	6 (23.1)	12 (30.0)	
	Obesity class 2	3 (4.5)	0 (0.0)	3 (7.5)	
	Obesity class 3	0 (0.0)	0 (0.0)	0 (0.0)	

Time × Group Interaction on Primary Outcomes Over Time

Results show that there were no statistically significant time × group interactions at any of the walking distances over the three assessment times. However, there was a significant main effect of time, with a large effect size, on PFWD [$F(2,54)$ = 38.05, $p < 0.001$, $\eta p^2 = 0.585$], FWD [$F(2,53) = 49.84$, $p < 0.001$, $\eta p^2 = 0.65$], MWD [$F(2,57) = 36.59$, $p < 0.001$, $\eta p^2 = 0.56$], and 6MWD [$F(2,57) = 15.34$, $p < 0.001$, $\eta p^2 = 0.35$].

Pairwise comparison showed: (A) an increased PFWD score between time 1 and time 3, from 123.76 to 307.66, respectively, with a difference of 183.58 metres (±185.46, 95% CI: 134.47–233.32 metres; $p < 0.05$), statistically significant in 6 months of the program. Differences were also found between time 1 and time 2 (161.36 ± 146.56, 95% CI: 118.24–194.79 metre; $p < 0.05$), but not between time 2 and time 3; (B) an increased FWD score between time 1 and time 3, from 191.70 to 398.75, respectively, with a difference of 206.6 metres (±173.34, 95% CI: 160.26–253.83 metres; $p < 0.05$) statistically significant in 6 months of the program. Differences were also found between time 1 and time 2 (188.1 ± 146.56, 95% CI: 141.57–225.09 metres; $p < 0.05$), but not between time 2 and time 3; (C) an increased MWD score between time 1 and time 3, from 311.50 to 541.30, respectively, with a difference of 229.80 metres (±223.96, 95% CI: 171.43–288.16 metres; $p < 0.05$), statistically significant in 6 months of the program. Differences were also found between time 1 and time 2 (193.43 ± 189.50, 95% CI: 144.12–242.74 metres; $p < 0.05$), but not between time 2 and time 3; (D) an increased 6MWT score between time 1 and time 3, from 335.73 to 378.54 metres, respectively, with a difference of 42.81 metres (±61.21, 95% CI: 26.85–58.76 metres; $p < 0.05$), statistically significant in 6 months of the program. Differences were also found between time 1 and time 2 (34.93 ± 60.03, 95% CI: 19.33–50.51 metres; $p < 0.05$), but not between time 2 and time 3.

Time × Group Interaction on Secondary Outcomes Over Time

A repeated-measures ANOVA, with a Greenhouse-Geisser correction, determined that: (A) the mean value of VascQuol-6 differed significantly across three time points ($F(2,57) = 23.60$, $p < 0.001$). Pairwise comparison showed an increased VascQuol-6 score between time 1 and time 3 (15.6 vs. 19.3, respectively), with a difference of 3.7 points (±4.20) statistically significant ($p < 0.05$). The differences were also statistically significant from time 1 to time 2 (1.8 ± 3.81, $p < 0.05$) and from time 2 to time 3 (1.9 ± 3.06 $p < 0.05$). Therefore, we can conclude that the ANOVA results indicate a significant effect of time on the QoL over the 6 months of the WalkingPad program; (B) the walking distance impairment score differed significantly across three time points ($F(2,57) = 56.99$, $p < 0.001$). Pairwise comparison showed an increase in walking distance ability between time 1 and time 3 (28.97 vs. 70.45, respectively), with a difference of 41.47 ± 35.23 statistically significant ($p < 0.05$). The differences were also statistically significant from time 1 to time 2 (44.77 ± 34.93, $p < 0.05$). However, the increase in WIQ-distance score from time 2 to time 3, did not reach significance when comparing the initial assessment to a second assessment. Therefore, we can conclude that the ANOVA results indicate a significant effect of time on the walking distance impairment in the first 3 months of the program; (C) determined that the mean value of WIQ-speed differed significantly across three time points ($F(2,57) = 37.07$, $p < 0.001$). Pairwise comparison showed an increased WIQ-speed score between time 1 and time 3 (20.62 vs. 40.73, respectively), with a difference of 20.11 ± 26.08, statistically significant ($p < 0.05$). The differences were also found between time 1 and time 2 (20.38 ± 18.98, $p < 0.05$) but not between time 2 and time 3, where the velocity decreased, although not significantly; (D) that the mean value of WIQ-stairs differed significantly across three time points ($F(2,57) = 12.88$, $p < 0.001$). Pairwise comparison showed an increased WIQ-stairs score between time 1 and time 3 (41.32 vs. 71.18, respectively), with a difference of 29.86 ± 45.24 statistically significant ($p < 0.05$). The differences were also found between time 1 and time 2 (19.24 ± 50.22, $p < 0.05$) and between time 2 and time 3 (10.63 ± 40.27, $p < 0.05$) (Table 8.2).

Discussion

The aim of the WalkingPad program was to assess whether using a smartphone app – the WalkingPad app – significantly improved walking distances, abilities, and patient-reported outcomes at 3 and 6 months, compared to a group of patients who did not use the smartphone app. The results showed that there were no differences between the groups in the primary and secondary outcomes. However, there were statistically significant differences between assessment moments but mainly from time 1 to time 2 (3 months).

Table 8.2. Change of Scores on Primary and Secondary Outcomes.

	Change Score ΔT1–T2 (*n* = 36)	Change Score ΔT2–T3 (*n* = 36)	Change Score ΔT1–T3 (*n* = 36)
Treadmill test			
PFWD: Pain-free walking distance (metres)	194.66 (149.24)	37.20 (167.20)	224.79 (201.10)
FWD: Functional walking distance (metres)	197.50 (162.29)	43.23 (183.70)	238.94 (194.87)
MWD: Maximal walking distance (metres)	207.50 (171.35)	47.42 (175.26)	254.92 (213.44)
6-Minutes Walk Test			
6MWD: 6-minute walking distance (metres)	33.76 (64.95)	11.26 (52.04)	45.01 (56.12)
VascuQoL			
QoL (0–24)	0.694 (3.62)	1.806 (2.78)	2.500 (4.04)
WIQ			
WIQ_d: Walking impairment distance (0–100%)	34.85 (34.98)	0.559 (29.11)	34.29 (36.04)
WIQ_sp: Walking impairment speed (0–100%)	14.79 (17.58)	−0.771 (22.73)	14.02 (25.99)
WIQ_s: Walking impairment stairs (0–100%)	0.115 (48.74)	14.70 (39.93)	−14.81 (46.23)

Note: T1: time 1= baseline; T2: time 2 = 3 months; T3: time 3 = 6 months; Δ: difference.

Our first hypothesis was not confirmed. Participants assigned to the EG showed no greater increase in MWD, PFWD, FWD, 6MWD, or QoL, and showed no reduction in walking impairments (distance, speed, and climbing stairs) when compared to participants assigned to the CG . It was expected that the EG would present better results for using an application that allowed monitoring, feedback, and provided support as if it were a 'walking buddy', as verified in other studies (Argent et al., 2018; Duscha et al., 2018; Fokkenrood et al., 2012; Khambati et al., 2017; Kim et al., 2021). However, this did not happen. Therefore, we expect that increasing the sample will enhance the power of the results.

Our second hypothesis was confirmed. There were statistically significant differences over time in primary and secondary outcomes. PFWD, FWD, MWD, and 6MWD increase especially between times 1 and 2 and times 1 and 3. It seems that between time 2 and time 3, the goal is to maintain and not progress. The differences found in this study in distance walking are well above those found in other studies that also used HBET (Golledge et al., 2019), suggesting that HBET programs are indeed effective in increasing the distance walked in the first 3 months and maintaining the results achieved at the end of 6 months (Bullard et al., 2019; Golledge et al., 2019).

Regarding secondary outcomes, QoL increased between times 1 and 2 and times 2 and 3, suggesting that the WalkingPad program's impact on QoL is progressive, reinforcing the need for maintenance and the added value of a 6 months program.

Regarding walking impairment assessed by the WIQ, the distance walked, and the walking speed increased from time 1 to time 2. This result is in agreement with the results of the maximal distance walked objectively measured in the treadmill test and in the 6MWT. However, the speed decreased from time 2 to time 3 although it did not prove to be significant. The ability to climb stairs increased from time 1 to time 2 and from time 2 to time 3, suggesting that this is a skill favoured with a 6 months program.

The QoL of PAD patients is significantly associated with claudication pain, walking distance, and stair climbing (Kim et al., 2021). Thus, as distances and walking skills increase, so does the QoL over the six months.

Conclusions

It can be concluded that the WalkingPad program was able to increase walking distances, enhance the QoL, and decrease walking impairment for a period of 6 months compared to baseline. WalkingPAD app provides a simple platform that is effective, useful, and appreciated by patients with PAD, with a high level of usability.

Suggested Teaching Assignments

A. What is the role of M-Health technology in the treatment of cardiovascular disease?
B. Will AI have a role in identifying the best patient-centred exercise program?

Recommended Readings

Veiga, C., Pedras, S., Oliveira, R., Paredes, H., & Silva, I. (2022, December). A systematic review on smartphone use for activity monitoring during exercise therapy in intermittent claudication. *Journal of Vascular Surgery*, 76(6),1734–1741. https://doi.org/10.1016/j.jvs.2022.04.045. PMID: 35709859

Thanigaimani, S., Jin, H., Silva, M. T., & Golledge, J. (2022, October 21). Network meta-analysis of trials testing if home exercise programs informed by wearables measuring activity improve peripheral artery disease related walking impairment. *Sensors (Basel)*, 22(20), 8070. https://doi.org/10.3390/s22208070. PMID: 36298419; PMCID: PMC9611238

Pinto, B., Correia, M. V., Paredes, H., & Silva, I. (2023). Detection of intermittent claudication from smartphone inertial data in community walks using machine learning classifiers. *Sensors*, 23(3), 1581. https://doi.org/10.3390/s23031581

Al-Ramini, A., Hassan, M., Fallahtafti, F., Takallou, M. A., Rahman, H., Qolomany, B., Pipinos, I. I., Alsaleem, F., & Myers, S. A. (2022). Machine learning-based peripheral artery disease identification using laboratory-based gait data. *Sensors*, 22, 7432. https://doi.org/10.3390/s22197432

Rodrigues, E., & Silva, I. (2020, February). Supervised exercise therapy in intermittent claudication: A systematic review of clinical impact and limitations. *Internation Angiology*, 39(1), 60–75. https://doi.org/10.23736/S0392-9590.19.04159-2. PMID: 31782277

Case study

Male, 65 years, Caucasian. Married. 2 sons.
Informatic Engineer
Cardiovascular risk factors present are heavy smoker, hypertension and high cholesterol levels since five years ago.
No other pathologies.
Family history of cardiovascular disease: mother died of stroke and grandfather died from heart attack.
Attending outpatient clinic due to pain in the legs when walking. He has no rest pain or trophic lesions.
Medication: aspirin 150 mg qd, losartan 50 mg qd, and atorvastatin 40 mg qd.
Clinically only femoral pulses are present. No lesion in the foot. Capillary refill 5 seconds.
A B/I: left 0.65; right 0.71.
Duplex scan: Triphasic curves at femoral arteries; remainder monophasic.
Treadmill test: stops at 200 metre due to leg pain.
6-Minutes walking test: pain at 170 metre.

Questions:

1. What would be first-line therapy for this patient?
2. How would you motivate this man to accomplish this treatment?
3. How could technology help you to implement this treatment program?

Titles for Research Essays

1. Home-based Exercise Therapy Versus Walking Advice for Intermittent Claudication
2. Wearable Activity Monitors in Home-based Exercise Therapy: Challenges
3. Role of Cognitive-Behavioural Techniques for the Management of Intermittent Claudication
4. Supervised Exercise Therapy Versus Non-supervised Exercise Therapy for Peripheral Arterial Disease

Recommended Projects URL

https://play.google.com/store/apps/details?id=walkingpad.distancepad
https://www.inesctec.pt/en/projects/walkingpad

References

Aboyans, V., Ricco, J. B., Bartelink, M. L. E. L., Björck, M., Brodmann, M., Cohnert, T., Collet, J.-P., Czerny, M., De Carlo, M., Debus, S., Espinola-Klein, C., Kahan, T., Kownator, S., Mazzolai, L., Naylor, A. R., Roffi, M., Röther, J., Sprynger, M., Tendera, M., Tepe, G., ... ESC Scientific Document Group. (2018). Editor's Choice – 2017 ESC guidelines on the diagnosis and treatment of peripheral arterial diseases, in collaboration with the European Society for Vascular Surgery (ESVS). *European Journal of Vascular and Endovascular Surgery, 55*(3), 305–368.

Anderson, J. D., Epstein, F. H., Meyer, C. H., Hagspiel, K. D., Wang, H., Berr, S. S., ... & Kramer, C. M. (2009). Multifactorial determinants of functional capacity in peripheral arterial disease: uncoupling of calf muscle perfusion and metabolism. *Journal of the American College of Cardiology, 54*(7), 628–635.

Argent, R., Daly, A., & Caulfield, B. (2018).Patient involvement with home-based exercise programs: Can connected health interventions influence adherence? *JMIR mHealth uHealth, 6*(3), e47.

Bohannon, R. W., & Magasi, S. (2015).Identification of dynapenia in older adults through the use of grip strength t-scores. *Muscle and Nerve, 51*(1), 102–105.

Bullard, T., Ji, M., An, R., Trinh, L., Mackenzie, M., & Mullen, S. P. (2019). A systematic review and meta-analysis of adherence to physical activity interventions among three chronic conditions: cancer, cardiovascular disease, and diabetes. *BMC public health, 19*(1), 1–11.

Correia, M.A., Andrade-Lima, A., Oliveira, P.L.M., Domiciano, R.M., Domingues, W.J.R., Wolosker, N., Puench-Leão, P., Ritti-Dias, R.M., & Cucato, G.G. (2018). Translation and Validation of the Brazilian-Portuguese Short Version of Vascular Quality of Life Questionnaire in Peripheral Artery Disease Patients with Intermittent Claudication Symptoms. *Annals of Vascular Surgery*, (51), 48–54, e1 https://doi.org/10.1016/j.avsg.2018.02.026.

Duscha, B. D., Piner, L. W., Patel, M. P., Crawford, L. E., Jones, W. S., Patel, M. R., & Kraus, W. E. (2018).Effects of a 12-week mHealth Program on functional capacity and physical activity in patients with peripheral artery disease. *American Journal of Cardiology [Internet], 122*(5), 879–884. https://doi.org/10.1016/j.amjcard.2018.05.018

Ekkekakis, P., & Dafermos, M. (2012). Exercise is a many-splendored thing, but for some it does not feel so splendid: Staging a resurgence of hedonistic ideas in the quest to understand exercise behavior. In P. E. Nathan & E. Acevedo (Eds.), *The Oxford handbook of exercise psychology* (pp. 295–333). Oxford University Press.

Ekkekakis, P. (2013). *The Measurement of Affect, Mood, and Emotion: A Guide for Health-Behavioral Research.* Cambridge: Cambridge University Press. https://doi.org/10.1017/CBO9780511820724

Fokkenrood, H. J. P., Lauret, G. J., Scheltinga, M. R. M., Spreeuwenberg, C., de Bie, R. A., & Teijink, J. A. W. (2012).Multidisciplinary treatment for peripheral arterial occlusive disease and the role of eHealth and mHealth. *Journal of Multidisciplinary Healthcare, 5,* 257–263.

Galea, M. N., Weinman, J. A., White, C., & Bearne, L. M. (2013). Do behavior-change techniques contribute to the effectiveness of exercise therapy in patients with intermittent claudication? A systematic review. *European Journal of Vascular and Endovascular Surgery, 46*(1), 132–141. https://doi.org/10.1016/j.ejvs.2013.03.030

Gaudreau, P., Carraro, N., & Miranda, D. (2012).From goal motivation to goal progress: The mediating role of coping in the self-concordance model. *Anxiety Stress Coping, 25*(5), 507–528.

Gerhard-Herman, M. D., Gornik, H. L., Barrett, C., Barshes, N. R., Corriere, M. A., Drachman D. E., Fleisher, L. A., Fowkes, F. G. R., Hamburg, N. M., Kinlay, S., Lookstein, R., Misra, S., Mureebe, L., Olin, J. W., Patel, R. A. G., Regensteiner, J. G., Schanzer, A., Shishehbor, M. H., Stewart, K. J., Treat-Jacobson, D., & Eileen Walsh, M. (2017).2016 AHA/ACC guideline on the management of patients with lower extremity peripheral artery disease: Executive summary: A report of the American college of cardiology/American Heart Association task force on clinical practice guidelines. *Circulation, 69*(11), e71–e126.

Golledge, J., Singh, T. P., Alahakoon, C., Pinchbeck, J., Yip, L., Moxon, J. V., & Morris, D. R. (2019).Meta-analysis of clinical trials examining the benefit of structured home exercise in patients with peripheral artery disease. *British Journal of Surgery, 106,* 319–331. https://doi.org/10.1002/bjs.11101

Harzand, A., Vakili, A. A., Alrohaibani, A., Abdelhamid, S. M., Gordon, N. F., Thiel, J., Benarroch-Gampel, J., Teodorescu, V. J., Minton, K., Wenger, N. K., Rajani, R. R., & Shah, A. J. (2020).Rationale and design of a smartphone-enabled, home-based exercise program in patients with symptomatic peripheral arterial disease: The smart step randomized trial. *Clinical Cardiology, 43*(6), 537–545. https://doi.org/10.1002/clc.23362

Henderson, L., Knight, T., & Richardson, B. (2013).An exploration of the wellbeing benefits of hedonic and eudaimonic behaviour. *The Journal of Positive Psychology, 8*(4), 322–336.

Khambati, H., Boles, K., & Jetty, P. (2017).Google Maps offers a new way to evaluate claudication. *Journal of Vascular Surgery, 65*(5), 1467–1472. http://dx.doi.org/10.1016/j.jvs.2016.11.047

Kim, K. S., Lee, S. J., & Suh, J. C. (1975).Mini-Mental State: A practical method for grading the cognitive state of patients for the clinician. *Journal of Psychiatric Research, 12*(3), 189–198.

Kim, M., Kim, C., Kim, E., & Choi, M. (2021). Effectiveness of mobile health–based exercise interventions for patients with peripheral artery disease: Systematic review and meta-analysis. *JMIR Mhealth Uhealth, 9*(2), e24080. https://doi.org/10.2196/24080

Kumlien, C., Nordanstig, J., Lundström, M., & Pettersson, M. (2017). Validity and test retest reliability of the vascular quality of life Questionnaire-6: a short form of a disease-specific health-related quality of life instrument for patients with peripheral arterial disease. *Health and Quality of Life Outcomes, 15*(1), 1–12.

Kruidenier, L. M., Nicolaï, S. P., Willigendael, E. M., de Bie, R. A., Prins, M. H, & Teijink, J. A. (2009).Functional claudication distance: A reliable and valid measurement to assess functional limitation in patients with intermittent claudication. *BMC Cardiovascular Disorder, 2*(9), 9. https://doi.org/10.1186/1471-2261-9-9. PMID: 19254382; PMCID: PMC2667172

Kwasnicka, D., Dombrowski, S. U., White, M., & Sniehotta, F. (2016). Theoretical explanations for maintenance of behaviour change: A systematic review of behaviour theories. *Health Psychology Review, 10*(3), 277–296. https://doi.org/10.1080/17437199.2016.1151372

McDermott, M. M., Greenland, P., Liu, K., Guralnik, J. M., Criqui, M. H., Dolan, N. C., ... & Martin, G. J. (2001). Leg symptoms in peripheral arterial disease: associated clinical characteristics and functional impairment. *Jama, 286*(13), 1599–1606.

McDermott, M. M. (2018).Exercise rehabilitation for peripheral artery disease. *Journal of Cardiopulmonary Rehabilitation and Prevention, 38*(2), 63–69. https://doi.org/ 10.1097/HCR.0000000000000343

Nicolaï, S. P. A., Kruidenier, L. M., Rouwet, E. V., Graffius, K., Prins, M. H., & Teijink, J. A. W. (2009).The Walking Impairment Questionnaire: An effective tool to assess the effect of treatment in patients with intermittent claudication. *Journal of Vascular Surgery [Internet], 50*(1), 89–94. http://dx.doi.org/10.1016/j.jvs.2008.12.073

Nordanstig, J., Wann-Hansson, C., Karlsson, J., Lundström, M., Pettersson, M., & Morgan, M. B. F. (2014).Vascular Quality of Life Questionnaire-6 facilitates health-related quality of life assessment in peripheral arterial disease. *Journal of Vascular Surgery [Internet], 59*(3), 700–707.e1. http://dx.doi.org/10.1016/j.jvs.2013.08.099

Norgren, L., Hiatt, W. R., Dormandy, J. A., Nehler, M. R., Harris, K. A., & Fowkes, F. G. R. (2007). Inter-Society consensus for the management of peripheral arterial disease (TASC II). *Journal of Vascular Surgery, 45*(Suppl 1), 5–67.

Parfitt, G., Rose, E. A., & Markland, D. (2000). The effect of prescribed and preferred intensity exercise on psychological affect and the influence of baseline measures of affect. *Journal of Health Psychology, 5*(2), 231–240.

Resnick, H. E., Lindsay, R. S., McDermott, M. M., Devereux, R. B., Jones, K. L., Fabsitz, R. R., & Howard, B. V. (2004). Relationship of high and low ankle brachial index to all-cause and cardiovascular disease mortality: the Strong Heart Study. *Circulation, 109*(6), 733–739.

Schulz, K. F., Altman, D. G., & Moher, D. (2010). CONSORT 2010 statement: updated guidelines for reporting parallel group randomised trials. *Journal of Pharmacology and pharmacotherapeutics, 1*(2), 100–107.

Segar, M. L., & Richardson, C. R. (2014). Prescribing pleasure and meaning: Cultivating walking motivation and maintenance. *American Journal of Preventive Medicine, 47*(6), 838–841. https://doi.org/10.1016/j.amepre.2014.07.001

Segar, M. L., Eccles, J. S., & Richardson, C. R. (2011).Rebranding exercise: Closing the gap between values and behavior. *International Journal of Behavioral Nutrition and Physical Activity, 8*, 94. https://doi.org/10.1186/1479-5868-8-94

Santulli, G., Shu, J. (2018). Update on peripheral artery disease: Epidemiology and evidence-based facts. *Atherosclerosis, 275*, 379–381.

Silva, I., Pedras, S., Oliveira, R., Veiga, C., & Paredes, H. (2022). WalkingPad protocol: A randomized clinical trial of behavioral and motivational intervention added to smartphone-enabled supervised home-based exercise in patients with peripheral arterial disease and intermittent claudication. *Trials, 23*, 326. https://doi.org/ 10.1186/s13063-022-06279-9

Striberger, R., Axelsson, M. Zarrouk, M., & Kumlien. C. (2020).Illness perceptions in patients with peripheral arterial disease – A systematic review of qualitative studies. *International Journal of Nursing Studies, 116*, 103723. https://doi.org/10.1016/j. ijnurstu.2020.103723

Teixeira, P. J., Carraça, E. V., Mariland, D., Silva, M. N., & Ryan, R. M. (2012). Exercise, physical activity, and self-determination theory: A systematic review. *The International Journal of Behavioral Nutrition and Physical Activity, 9*, 78. https://doi. org/10.1186/1479-5868-9-78

Treat-Jacobson, D., McDermott, M. M., Beckman, J. A., Burt, M. A., Creager, M. A., Ehrman, J. K., Gardner, A. W., Mays, R. J., Regensteiner, J. G., Salisbury, D. L., Schorr, E. N., & Walsh, M. E. (2019).Implementation of supervised exercise therapy for patients with symptomatic peripheral artery disease: A Science Advisory from the American Heart Association. *Circulation, 140*(13), E700–E710.

Chapter 9

Chronic Pain and Strategies to Improve Patient Health

Raul Marques Pereira[a,b,c]

[a]*Unidade Local de Saúde do Alto Minho, Viana do Castelo, Portugal*
[b]*School of Medicine, Minho University, Braga, Portugal*
[c]*P5 Digital Medical Center, Minho University, Braga, Portugal*

Abstract

The process of chronic pain (CP) and strategies is to improve the patient's health and well-being. CP is a frequent medical problem that presents a major challenge to healthcare providers because of its complex natural history, imprecise aetiology, and inadequate response to pharmacological treatment. Although different definitions exist it is widely accepted that CP is an ongoing pain that lasts more than 3 months or that persists longer than the reasonably expected healing time for the involved tissues. Also, it is acknowledged that its treatment is much different than the treatment for acute pain. When addressing a person with CP, one should always keep in mind that pain is much more about the individual than the underlying medical condition. Every person is different, and healthcare providers should take a tailor-made approach to managing their pain. This is the only way to ensure good results in pain treatment. Treatment goals should be discussed and adapted to the patient profile. It is fundamental to have clear goals from the beginning and to ensure these are realistic, individualized, and measurable. Effective treatment for CP is only achieved through a holistic framework in which the patient's well-being is the first concern and an interdisciplinary and societal approach is implemented from the first day.

Keywords: Chronic pain; holistic; well-being; individualized; interdisciplinary; health literacy

Technology-Enhanced Healthcare Education:
Transformative Learning for Patient-Centric Health, 115–127
Copyright © 2024 by Raul Marques Pereira
Published under exclusive licence by Emerald Publishing Limited
doi:10.1108/978-1-83753-598-920231009

What Is Pain?

The International Association for the Study of Pain (IASP) introduced since 1979, a revised definition of pain by Raja et al. (2020) bring the result of a two-year process that the association hopes will lead to revised ways of assessing pain.

This revised definition intends to better convey the nuances and the complexity of pain lead to improved assessment and management of those with pain.

The definition is: 'An unpleasant sensory and emotional experience associated with, or resembling that associated with, actual or potential tissue damage', and is expanded upon by the addition of six key notes and the etymology of the word pain for further valuable context:

- Pain is always a personal experience that is influenced to varying degrees by biological, psychological, and social factors.
- Pain and nociception are different phenomena. Pain cannot be inferred solely from activity in sensory neurons.
- Through their life experiences, individuals learn the concept of pain.
- A person's report of an experience is pain should be respected.
- Although pain usually serves an adaptive role, it may have adverse effects on function and social and psychological well-being.
- Verbal description is one of the several behaviours to express pain; the inability to communicate does not negate the possibility that a human or a non-human animal experiences pain.

This revised definition was developed by a multinational, multidisciplinary Task Force with input from all potential stakeholders, including persons in pain and their caregivers.

Pain can be anything from slightly bothersome, such as a mild headache, to something excruciating and emergent, such as the chest pain that accompanies a heart attack, or pain of kidney stones. Pain can be acute, meaning new, subacute, lasting for a few weeks or months, and chronic, when it lasts for more than 3 months.

CP is long-standing pain that persists beyond the usual recovery period or occurs along with a chronic health condition, such as arthritis. CP may be 'on' and 'off' or continuous. It may affect people to the point that they can't work, eat properly, take part in physical activity, or enjoy life.

CP is one of the costliest health problems in the United States. Increased medical expenses, lost income, lost productivity, compensation payments, and legal charges are some of the economic consequences of CP (Dagenais, 2008).

CP is a major medical condition as shown in Fig. 9.1 that can and should be treated.

Patients' View on CP Care – Impact Considerations

Studies performed in different settings have demonstrated that CP affects between 10% and 30% of the adult population in Europe. CP interferes with different

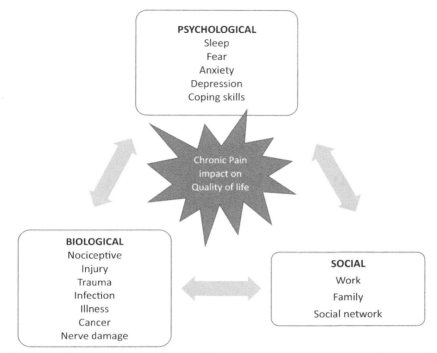

Fig. 9.1.   Biopsychosocial Model of Pain and Consequences on the Quality of Life. *Source*: Adapted from María Dueñas (2016).

aspects of the patient's life, negatively affecting their daily activities, physical and mental health, family and social relationships, and their interactions in the workplace. It also affects the healthcare system and what is known as economic well-being, the strong burden associated with CP not only derives from healthcare costs but also from the loss of productivity and from payments to patients as a result of the disability that pain produces (María Dueñas, 2016).

Repercussions on Bodily Functions and Daily Routines

Several research papers have examined the impact of CP on the lives of patients, demonstrating the association between this condition and limited physical activity.

Intensity, duration, and location of pain have a decisive effect on a patient's physical performance, reducing their physical activity, and even producing impairment, which impacts other facets of their daily lives (Jones et al., 2008).

In a survey conducted throughout Europe, the majority of individuals with CP suffered from a variety of limitations, with the ability to perform intense physical exercise, walk, perform household chores, participate in social activities, and maintain an independent lifestyle being the most affected (Amris et al., 2011).

CP sufferers, in contrast to pain-free persons, are frequently unaware of their degree of physical activity, as objective and subjective measurements of their physical activity differ.

This is intriguing because, if patients overestimate their level of activity, they may conclude that it is sufficient and lose the desire or drive to modify their behaviour and increase their activity. The intention or motive to change is one of the most important determinants of behavioural changes, according to conventional theoretical models. This is why making patients aware of their behaviour can increase the likelihood that they choose a healthier lifestyle, become more active, and have less pain-related incapacity (Langley et al., 2011).

Health-related Quality of Life Effects

The patient's mental and physical quality of life is another indicator of the harmful effects of pain. Several studies conducted on patients with fibromyalgia, rheumatoid arthritis, or low back pain have shown that these conditions frequently cause a significant decline in the patient's quality of life (Carmona et al., 2001).

Some correlations between pain intensity and quality of life scores have been identified in pain sufferers, indicating that the more intense the pain, the poorer the quality of life. In addition, individuals with severe and frequent pain have a lower quality of life than those with moderate and less frequent pain, because their pain has a higher influence on the physical dimensions than the mental ones. In contrast, pain severity, anxiety or depression symptoms, and emotion-focused coping techniques were the factors that had the greatest impact on the quality of life of fibromyalgia patients (Campos & Rodríguez, 2012).

CP patients frequently report sleep difficulties, which are intimately related to quality of life. Sleep difficulties may increase stress levels, and as a result, such disturbances can make it difficult for patients to do simple tasks and may even damage their cognitive abilities, so reducing their ability to carry out routine chores at work and at home (Tüzün, 2007).

Work-related Repercussions

The impact of pain in work is a crucial consideration for CP patients. Studies conducted in several nations have demonstrated that pain-affected people have absenteeism issues. As a result of their pain symptoms, not only are they frequently required to change their job responsibilities or position, but they may also lose their employment (Azevedo et al., 2012).

Other research papers have also demonstrated that CP-related absenteeism, presenteeism, early retirement, and disability present a burden comparable to those of typically highlighted public health issues. When analyzing the occupational effects of various types of pain, backache, and rheumatic disease-related pain created the most days of sick leave, respectively. Neuropathic pain may also negatively impact work performance and increase absenteeism, resulting in decreased productivity and an inability to meet certain duties. It is difficult for patients to maintain a normal lifestyle in light of these consequences in the workplace (Breivik, 2013).

In patients with low back pain, notably, those aged 45–65, it has been found that low back pain is one of the most often mentioned medical reasons for work loss. In addition, it has been demonstrated that even though 20% of adults of working age seek medical attention and only 20% record illness absence due to back discomfort, this tiny number accounts for the majority of these individuals' healthcare costs and socioeconomic burden. Similarly, it has been demonstrated that between 43% and 78% of fibromyalgia patients are on sick leave, and that their total disability status ranges from 6.7% to 30% (Costa-Black et al., 2010).

CP patient relatives may share and reinforce certain emotions, such as a fear of pain or the development of a new work-related injury, and they may be pessimistic about the patient's ability to return to work. In certain instances, family members are resigned to the bad effects that backache has on occupational activity, and they harbour skepticism regarding the prospect of finding a position suited to the patient's needs and/or an accommodating attitude on the part of superiors. Notably, instead of focusing solely on individual risk factors linked with long-term absenteeism, it is vital to assess how the patient's social environment and the people around him or her may contribute to the onset or persistence of pain, as well as its repercussions.

Social and Familial Repercussions

CP can also have an impact on a patient's social interactions, limiting their leisure activities and social engagements. Indeed, a large number of patients with pain say that their condition prohibits them from attending social or family events, and similarly, have decreased family interaction.

Studies on people with osteoarthritis or fibromyalgia indicate that physical and mental issues, as well as pain, have a major impact on social functioning. Similarly, a loss in physical capacity and mental health has been found in neuropathic pain patients, which significantly contributes to their impaired social integration. Additionally, the negative emotions, impatience, and hostility that frequently characterize these patients have a deleterious effect on interpersonal interactions and family stress levels (Hill et al., 1999).

The incapacity caused by pain and the dependence it frequently induces can also have repercussions for the individual's family and acquaintances. In particular, family members are frequently required to perform tasks such as caregiving, supervision, participation in and evaluation of therapies, and involvement in decision-making when consulting physicians. Relatives may experience physical and psychological decline as a result of these new responsibilities, which they frequently find difficult to manage: feelings of melancholy, being overloaded, frustration, and helplessness. Indeed, these family members' social, professional, and daily lives are also significantly impacted (Bigatti & Cronan, 2002).

Several studies that studied the impact of oncological and non-oncological pain on relatives who serve as caretakers discovered that more than 30% of those polled stated they were unable to cope with the pain-related issues impacting their relatives. Many of them experienced anxiety and depression, and depression in the caregiver was associated with a patient's greater pain intensity.

Intriguingly, from a neurological standpoint, there is a connection between a pain-stricken individual and the surroundings, notably the family or relatives. For instance, seminal research from Mogil's group in Montreal has proved conclusively that this influence may be linked to the phenomena of empathy (Mogil, 2015). In reality, it appears that some regions of the central nervous system are involved in this process, namely the amygdala, insula, and anterior cingulate cortex. These regions are represented in the 'pain matrix' (Price, 2002).

Health Literacy and Patient Education – Considerations for Patient Centric Care

Evidence points to a critical role of self-management in reaching or maintaining better health outcomes in people with chronic conditions (Kima et al., 2022).

To encourage self-management abilities, one must equip the patient with knowledge and skills matched with his or her beliefs and preferences, such as problem-solving strategies.

Individual and Family Self-Management Theory (IFSMT) provides complete guidance for explaining pain and its impact on function through self-management context-specific elements and processes among tested self-management models. The IFSMT postulates that contextual elements of self-management, such as the individual's perception of pain conditions, influence self-management processes, such as self-regulation, therefore influencing self-management behaviours and pain. IFSMT correlations between psychosocial process factors, self-management behaviours, and outcomes have been validated (Lucas et al., 2019; Verchota & Sawin, 2016).

Health literacy has emerged as a self-management factor. The US Institute of Medicine's definition, capacities to obtain, process, and comprehend information and services necessary for making health decisions provides a conceptual basis for identifying functionally health illiterate patients, so that clinicians can tailor communication strategies (Nutbeam, 2015).

In the meantime, the World Health Organization's definition of health literacy, the cognitive and social abilities that define an individual's motivation and ability to obtain, interpret, and apply health information to maintain good health, corresponds with an asset model for health literacy. In addition to to functional literacy, this asset-based approach includes communicative and critical literacy, which entails deriving meaning from diverse communication formats and evaluating the trustworthiness and dependability of information, respectively.

In the asset approach, health literacy can be increased by education and leads to better self-management outcomes, such as participation in pain self-management and less pain.

Pain Self-management

Typically, the term 'pain self-management strategies' refers to the measures an individual employs to reduce the impact of pain on their everyday lives, mood, and functions (e.g. sleep), whether at home or at work (Nicholas & Blyth, 2016).

This may be compared to the actions of a person could take to mitigate the damage caused by a hurricane. Although the person may not be able to manage the storm itself, there are numerous things she/he can take to mitigate its impact. The word self-management suggests that the individual in issue is taking an active part; they are doing something that has the potential to affect outcomes. However, various words have been used to define this job, which can make it difficult to comprehend the literature (Michie et al., 2011).

The issue of definitions is neither minor nor limited to the literature on pain. In reference to behaviour change approaches, in general, the absence of uniformity and clarity in these criteria makes it difficult to compare and evaluate ostensibly different methods, or even to combine methods that use the same term but are substantively distinct.

In numerous research, 'self-help' has referred to the acquisition of self-management skills or tactics. When a person with pain attempts to learn how to manage their symptoms without direct professional support, this is commonly referred to as 'self-administered' or 'unguided' self-care. This may be accomplished, for instance, through a brochure or a website. However, when direct professional aid is provided in learning self-management, this is typically referred to as 'guided self-help'. Less obvious is the distinction between guided self-help and psychologically based interventions such as cognitive behavioural therapy (CBT) (Berger et al., 2011).

Consequently, guided self-help for CP that utilizes CBT techniques and CBT for CP might be deemed equivalent. The only difference may be the treatment's duration or the number of sessions (in other words: brief CBT or extended CBT).

A Tailor-made Approach for the Treatment of CP

Patients with CP contact a healthcare professional three times as often as the overall adult population, on average 12 times over the course of 6 months. Most receive their initial consultation with a general practitioner, but only 1 in 5 feel hopeful about their CP after this consultation. In Europe, only 2% of patients with CP report being managed by a pain specialist, even though 68% of respondents to one survey were still in pain for more than 12 hours per day despite treatment, and 95% of patients in another survey supported by European Pain Federation (EFIC) and the World Institute of Pain remained in moderate or severe pain one year after the beginning of treatment (Kress et al., 2015).

There is an urgent need for physicians to communicate the biopsychosocial nature of CP and the significance of its psychological component, as well as the evidence that addressing the underlying disease generally results in pain relief. The issue of inadequate physician–patient communication reduces the probability of forming a shared understanding of the patient's condition and establishing reasonable treatment expectations. In relation to the degree of pain, effective communication is of utmost importance, although a survey of over 1,000 primary care practitioners (PCP) in 13 European countries revealed that only 48% employed pain assessment instruments, principally visual analogue scales and numerical rating scales. Even when these techniques are utilized, the outcomes are frequently not recorded in patients' medical records (Johnson et al., 2013).

In the majority of European nations, pain medicine is neither a speciality nor a sub-specialty; hence, the qualifications and definition of a pain specialist remain arbitrary and vague. This condition must be accepted due to the continued absence of broadly agreed curriculum for pain medicine education. In spite of this, there are physicians who specialize in pain medicine, and their discontent with the therapy of chronic non-cancer pain in Europe is well-documented.

Few resources are dedicated towards CP prevention and delivering effective treatment that follows established patient pathways based on best practice models, according to a substantial number of primary care professionals. Also, early diagnosis and management are essential, but the lack of training among non-specialists implies that acute pain is frequently not optimally treated and leads to CP, which is also improperly diagnosed and managed (Kehlet et al., 2006).

Pain specialists mostly blame inadequate care to non-adherence to evidence-based treatment, sub-optimal prescribing, and a dearth of viable medicines for complex and mixed pain syndromes. Although many patients with CP are treated in general practice – and this will continue – the situation is exacerbated by a widespread shortage of pain specialists in most countries and psychologists, as well as the absence of evidence-based practical guidelines for managing different types of chronic non-cancer pain.

Due to the multimodal, biopsychosocial nature of CP, all applicable modes of intervention are necessary for its prevention and treatment. Even though the biopsychosocial model of pain strongly suggests that somatic and psychological therapies should be administered simultaneously, integrating psychological therapy is rarely considered until pharmacological treatment has failed to provide adequate pain relief – which is too late for many patients. This may be partially due to the fact that few clinical or health psychologists are now employed in the primary care of pain patients, as well as the fact that physicians are not completely aware of the benefits of psychological treatment in managing CP. In addition, many patients may be resistant to acknowledge the importance of psychological therapy in the development of coping techniques, perceiving it as a personal failure that shows their agony is 'all in their head' (Kress et al., 2015).

In contrast, some psychologists may not pay enough attention to the bodily aspect of therapy. In addition, some guidelines do not specify which psychological interventions should be evaluated for which specific problems, while others are inapplicable to contemporary interventions utilizing a biopsychosocial approach. There is a need for high-quality, evidence-based guidelines that give a more comprehensive, biopsychosocial approach and provide guidance on the appropriate format, content, and length of such treatment.

A Multidisciplinary Pain Program, Technologically Enhanced, as a Process to High-value Care

A good example of a Multidisciplinary Pain Program is the Veterans Health Administration (VA) pain program (Aram & Mardian, 2020; Department of Veterans Affairs & Department of Defense, 2017). This pain program is a good illustration of a pain treatment system meant to provide high-value pain care and shut the evidence practice gap by using the sociopsychobiological (SPB) model.

The Chronic Pain Wellness Center (CPWC) of the Phoenix VA Health Care System was established in 2013 as a highly integrated interprofessional team providing pain and opioid use disorder treatment to US veterans. Existing literature documents the clinical effectiveness and cost-effectiveness of interdisciplinary pain care as used by the CPWC in a variety of domains, including pain severity, disability, pain self-efficacy, mood, pain-related anxiety, healthcare utilization, amount of medication used, and the sustainability of gains over a one-year follow-up (Kamper et al., 2014).

Over the past decade, the VA has worked to implement SPB pain treatment and increase access to interdisciplinary pain rehabilitation programs and alternative and integrative health providers, described in Fig. 9.2.

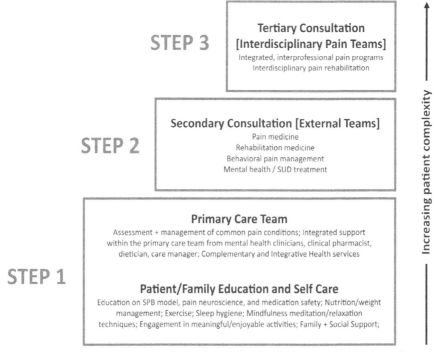

Fig. 9.2. Contemporary Example of an Effective SPB Implementation of Interprofessional Pain Treatment.
This figure illustrates the relationship of a pain care system within the larger healthcare system. As patient complexity, risk, and comorbidity increase, the therapeutic approach and the care setting become progressively more intensive. SPB, sociopsychobiological model; SUD, substance use disorder.
Source: Adapted from Veterans Affairs/Department of Defense Stepped Care Model of Pain Care (Department of Veterans Affairs & Department of Defense, 2017).

The primary care team delivers comprehensive, longitudinal, and progressive pain management with a focus on functional rehabilitation. Through the consultation process, the PCP can directly access a variety of specialty care services for patients with CP and pain-related comorbidities for patients with low-to-moderate complexity. Physical therapy, recreational therapy (includes adaptive exercise, yoga, tai chi, and core-strengthening classes), mental health services (which are both embedded within primary care for lower-complexity patients and available through the general mental health clinic for higher-complexity patients), CBT for chronic pain, and group auricular acupuncture paired with health coaching are among the specialty referrals directly available to the PCP. The goal of PCPs is to identify the subset of patients having evidence-based justifications for interventional pain procedures so that these patients can be referred directly for interventional procedures.

The PCP refers veterans with severe CP to the CPWC for evaluation and treatment suggestions.

The CPWC's initial patient evaluation is intended to promote high-quality care. Entry into many pain clinics is performed by an interventional pain physician, which likely results in earlier use of interventional pain procedures and broader implementation of these procedures.

In contrast, to facilitate a self-management approach that favours evidence-based active therapies, a primary care pain physician (PCPP) serves as the CPWC's entry point. A PCPP is an internist or family physician with additional training in pain management and/or addiction medicine. The PCPP produces a comprehensive care plan that emphasizes active therapies and serves as a treatment plan for the long term. According to the value continuum, passive therapy are prioritized, and interventional pain procedures are reserved for a subset of patients with evidence-based indications. Interventional pain techniques are also used wisely to reduce dependency on these operations or to reduce the usage of other high-risk medicines (e.g. high-dose opioid therapy). For more complex pain situations with greater psychosocial complexity, the CPWC entry point will be a co-disciplinary consultation with a PCPP and a pain psychologist. The initial visit permits a comprehensive SPB assessment, in addition to other care criteria (e.g. red flags review, physical examination, suicide risk assessment, mental health screening, etc.). Within the first few appointments, a plan of treatment tailored to the individual's specific SPB needs is devised.

Before their intake appointment with a PCPP, the majority of new patients referred to the CPWC will attend a group education class that includes basic pain neuroscience education, opioid safety principles, and a review of treatment options available. This is done in order to maximize the efficiency of the intake visit.

Implementing this Stepped Care Model outside an integrated healthcare system presents a number of obstacles. Worldwide low levels of investment in primary care resources are one of the obstacles to implementation. Moreover, it is regrettable that team-based pain care is uncommon in healthcare settings outside integrated healthcare systems like the VA. Innovative and novel procedures are urgently required to establish efficient ways to provide multimodal team-based pain care in a variety of contexts, particularly the early administration of movement and mental health therapies to patients at risk of developing high-impact CP.

Conclusion

The fundamental discussion of effective strategies for improving patient's health in CP arises from the need of a multidimensional approach to pain care from the moment of diagnosis.

Only through a stepped but robust care beginning in a primary care setting will it be possible to improve our quality of care and minimize the progression for severe CP.

Learning Sections

1. *Suggested teaching assignments*:

   o Search the internet, for example, of chronic pain protocols in primary care
   o develop a SWOT analysis.

2. Recommended readings:

   o https://www.changepain.com/about-us
   o https://www.changepain.com/change-your-pain/caregivers-guide
   o https://www.iasp-pain.org/education/online-learning-perc/

3. *Case study*:

   o Discuss the following clinical a situation: a young man with chronic low back pain, unable to work for 3 months while awaiting surgery
   o discuss the medical, psychological, and societary impact of this chronic pain condition.

4. Recommended Projects URL:

   o https://www.changepain.com
   o https://www.iasp-pain.org/
   o https://europeanpainfederation.eu/
   o https://apmgf.pt/grupos_de_estudo/dor/ (in portuguese)

References

Amris, K., Wæhrens, E. E., Jespersen, A., Bliddal, H., Danneskiold-Samsøe, B. (2011). Observation-based assessment of functional ability in patients with chronic widespread pain: A cross-sectional study. *Pain*, *152*(11), 2470–2476.

Aram, S., & Mardian, M. E.-R. (2020). Flipping the pain care model: A sociopsychobiological approach to high-value chronic pain care. *Pain Medicine*, *21*(6), 1168–1180.

Azevedo, L. F., Costa-Pereira, A., Mendonça, L., Dias, C. C., & Castro-Lopes, J. M. (2012). Epidemiology of chronic pain: A population-based nationwide study on its prevalence, characteristics and associated disability in Portugal. *Journal of Pain*, *13*(8), 773–783.

Berger, T., Hämmerli, K., Gubser, N., Andersson, G., & Caspar, F. (2011). Internet-based treatment of depression: A randomized controlled trial comparing guided with unguided self-help. *Cognitive Behavioral Therapy*, *40*(4), 251–266.

Bigatti, S. M., & Cronan, T. A. (2002). An examination of the physical health, h. u.-b. *Health Psychology*, *21*(2), 157–166.

Breivik, H. E. E. (2013). The individual and societal burden of chronic pain in Europe: The case for strategic prioritisation and action to improve knowledge and availability of appropriate care. *BMC Public Health*, 13, 1229.

Campos, R. P., & Rodríguez, M. I. V. (2012). Health-related quality of life in women with fibromyalgia: Clinical and psychological factors associated. *Clinical Rheumatology*, *31*(2), 347–355.

Carmona, L., Ballina, J., Gabriel, R., Laffon, A., &EPISER Study Group. (2001). The burden musculoskeletal diseases in the general population of Spain: Results from a national survey. *Annals of Rheumatolgy Disease*, *60*(11), 1040–1045.

Costa-Black, K. M., Loisel, P., Anema, J. R., & Pransky, G. (2010). Back pain and work. *Best Practices Research Rheumatology*, *24*(2), 227–240.

Dagenais, S. C. (2008). A systematic review of low back pain cost of illness studies in the United States and internationally. *The Spine Journal*, *8*(1), 8–20.

Department of Veterans Affairs & Department of Defense. (2017). *VA/DoD clinical practice guideline for management of opioid therapy for chronic pain*. The Opioid Therapy for Chronic Pain Work Group.

Hill, C. L., Parsons, J., Taylor, A., & Leach, G. (1999). Health related quality of life in a population sample with arthritis. *Journal of Rheumatology*, *26*(9), 2029–2035.

Johnson, M., Collett, B., & Castro-Lopes, J. M. (2013). The challenges of pain management in primary care: a pan-European survey. *Journal of Pain Research*, *22*(6), 393–401.

Jones, J. R., Rutledge, D. N., Jones, K. D., Matallana, L., & Rooks, D. S. (2008). Self-assed physical function levels of women with fibromyalgia: A national survey. *Womens Health Issues*, *18*(5), 406–412.

Kamper, S, J., Apeldoorn, A. T., Chiarotto, A., Smeets, R. J. E. M., Ostelo, R. W. J. G., Guzman, J., & van Tulder, M. W. (2014). Multidisciplinary biopsychosocial rehabilitation for chronic low back pain. *Cochrane Database of Systematic Reviews*, *9*, CD000963.

Kehlet, H., Jensen, T. S., & Woolf, C. J. (2006). Persistent postsurgical pain: Risk factors and prevention. *Lancet*, *367*(9522), 1618–1625.

Kima, K., Yang, Y., Wang, Z., Chen, J., Barandouzi, Z. A., Hong, H., Han, H.-R., & Starkweather, A. (2022). A systematic review of the association between health literacy and pain self-management. *Patient Education and Counseling*, *105*(6), 1427–1440.

Kress, H.-G., Aldington, D., Alon, E., Coaccioli, S., Collett, B., Coluzzi, F., Huygen, F., Jaksch, W., Kalso, E., Kocot-Kępska, M., Mangas, A. C., Ferri, C. M., Mavrocordatos, P., Morlion, B., Müller-Schwefe, G., Nicolaou, A., Hernández, C. P., & Sichère, P. (2015). A holistic approach to chronic pain management that involves all stakeholders: Change is needed. *Current Medical Research and Opinion*, *31*(9), 1743–1754.

Langley, P. C., Ruiz-Iban, M. A., Molina, J. T., De Andres, J., & Castellón, J. R. G.-E. (2011). The prevalence, correlates and treatment of pain in Spain. *Journal of Medical Economics*, *14*(3), 367–380.

Lucas, R., Zhang, Y., Walsh, S. J., Evans, H., Young, E., & Starkweather, A. (2019). Efficacy of a breastfeeding pain self-management intervention: A pilot randomized controlled trial. *Nursing Research*, *68*(2), E1–E10.

María Dueñas, B. O. (2016). A review of chronic pain impact on patients, their social environment and the health care system. *Journal of Pain Research*, 457–467.

Michie, S., Williams, S., Sniehotta, F. F., & Dombrowski, S. U. (2011). A refined taxonomy of behaviour change techniques to help people change their physical activity and healthy eating behaviours: The CALO-RE taxonomy. *Psychology and Health, 26*(11), 1479–1498.

Mogil, J. S. (2015). Social modulation of and by pain in humans and rodents. *Pain, 156*(Suppl 1), S35–S41.

Nicholas, M. K., & Blyth, F. M. (2016). Are self-management strategies effective in chronic pain treatment? *Pain Management, 6*(1), 75–88.

Nutbeam, D. (2015). Defining, measuring and improving health literacy. *Health Evaluation and Promotion, 42*(4), 450–456.

Price, D. D. (2002). Central neural mechanisms that interrelate sensory and affective dimensions of pain. *Molecular Interventions, 2*(6), 392–403.

Raja, S. N., Carr, D. B., Cohen, M., Finnerup, N. B., Flor, H., Gibson, S., Keefe, F. J., Mogil, J. S., Ringkamp, M., Sluka, K. A., Song, X.-J., Stevens, B., Sullivan, M. D., Tutelman, P. R., Ushida, T., & Vader, K. (2020). The revised International Association for the Study of Pain definition of pain: Concepts, challenges, and compromises. *Pain, 161*(9), 1976–1982.

Tüzün, E. H. (2007). Quality of life in chronic musculoskeletal pain. *Best Practice & Research: Clinical Rheumatology, 21*(3), 567–579.

Verchota, G., & Sawin, K. J. (2016). Testing components of a self-management theory in adolescents with type 1 diabetes mellitus. *Nursing Research, 65*(6), 487–495.

Chapter 10

ACP Model – Assertiveness, Clarity, and Positivity: The Competencies of the New Era

Cristina Vaz de Almeida

PhD Communication Sciences, Health Literacy ISCSP-CAPP, Lisbon, Portugal

Abstract

In an era where health professionals are increasingly demanding, and communicative skills are one of the keys to improve the relationship with the patient. The communicative competencies of assertiveness, clarity in verbal and non-verbal language, and positivity, based on the positive construction of the patient's health path, improve the therapeutic relationship, as well as the relationship between professionals in the world of health complexity. The ACP Model is validated with extensive application by hundreds of professionals in Portugal who use it daily. Active learning is one of the most effective means of raising awareness and involving the professionals who are learning and implementing the ACP Model.

Keywords: Health literacy; assertiveness; clarity; plain language; positivity; health education

Introduction

Patients take appointments with various levels of education and health literacy, and, mostly, they do not understand what the professional tells them. Communication between them is a factor of great imbalance, leading to a lack of understanding and memorization of health instructions.

The origin and language used by the patient also have effects on their understanding of health instructions (Schriver et al., 2010; Watson, 2019).

Technology-Enhanced Healthcare Education:
Transformative Learning for Patient-Centric Health, 129–144
Copyright © 2024 by Cristina Vaz de Almeida
Published under exclusive licence by Emerald Publishing Limited
doi:10.1108/978-1-83753-598-920231010

Health has, however, a more desired goal, for the patient to make appropriate decisions about health care, to have adherence (Miller, 2016; Sørensen et al., 2012) and know how to act on health information. Since this does not happen and memory fails (Miller, 2016), the results show more hospitalizations (Espanha & Ávila, 2016), more premature deaths (Sabia et al., 2010; Sørensen et al., 2012), more emergency responses, and less prevention through screening (Sørensen et al., 2012).

Health professionals' communication competencies can decide patients' well-being (Vaz de Almeida & Belim, 2021). The health professional is the strongest element in the therapeutic relationship (Vaz de Almeida, 2018), through the requirement of a competent communication practice, so that patients can adopt healthy recommendations and behaviours (Koh et al., 2013) and can contribute more in solving the problems (Kim & Grunig, 2011).

ACP Model: Interdependent and Aggregate Use of Three Key Communication Skills

Communication is the heart of literacy. It is through communication that we make ourselves understood and understand others in this complex world, which becomes even more complex when we need to deal with health or lack thereof.

Health literacy is linked to literacy and involves people's knowledge, motivation, and skills to access, understand, evaluate, and apply health information in order to form judgements and make daily decisions about health care, disease prevention, and health promotion, to maintain or improve the quality of life (Sørensen et al., 2012).

The ACP Model resulted from a cross-sectional investigation, carried out with a sample of 484 health professionals (doctors and nurses), with a quantitative and qualitative approach, gathered by a mixed method.

The results showed, through 484 voices of health professionals, 88 of which were participants in 14 focus groups, 389 respondents in the Q-COM-LIT survey, and 7 interviews with qualified informants, that: (1) the assertive, clear, and positive language used in the therapeutic relationship contributes to increase the patient's understanding, in view of the guidance given to him/her by the health professional; (2) health professionals consider these communication skills an indispensable condition to improve the therapeutic relationship, to reduce concerted efforts to ensure the understanding of the patient, so that, when understanding the health instructions, optimize their therapeutic adherence, thus competing to increase the quality of health care and the improvement of health literacy of the patient and the system (Vaz de Almeida, 2020, p. 260).

ACP Model: Starting With Assertiveness

Respect between the parties balances interpersonal relationships. Assertiveness is an important ingredient for initiating, maintaining, and restoring balance in a relationship, particularly in health.

Alberti and Emmons (1976) define assertiveness as behaviour that allows a person to act in his best interest, defend himself without undue anxiety, express his rights without jeopardizing the rights of others (p. 2), make use of his emotional intelligence (Morris & Keltner, 2000; Stein & Book, 2006), and creating habits (learning) to express his feelings. Assertiveness means having respect for the others, for us, and demanding respect for yourself.

At the heart of interpersonal relationships, no one should place themselves above the other, despite the social advantages (Alberti & Emmons, 2008, p. 2), with a tacit goal of realizing the personal rights of each participant. However, because it is a complex relationship, in which the professional dominates a technical jargon that the patient may not understand, the 'strongest side of the balance plate' (Almeida, 2018, p. 33; Coombs & Ersser, 2004) must balance and establish a platform of equality in every interaction with the patient.

There is a set of theories that robustly support the use of assertiveness in balanced interpersonal relationships (Chart 10.1).

Assertiveness is also a component of the patient's participation in therapeutic interaction, where he expresses an opinion, expresses his preference, offers a suggestion or recommendation, reveals disagreement or some other challenge to the health professional, or makes a request (Cegala, 2011, p. 428).

Chart 10.1.   Some Theories That Support Therapeutic Assertiveness.

Theories to Sustain Therapeutic Assertiveness		
Theory and Authors	**Synthesis**	**Behaviours and Attitudes**
Relational theory Bruning and Ledingham (1998)	Promoting mutually beneficial, symmetrical interpersonal relationships that generate trust, commitment, and investment	Direct relationship, 'eyes in the eyes' Respectful Equitable Symmetric Reliable generator Commitment part of the party
Problem Solving Theory Kim and Grung (2011)	In the therapeutic relationship, the patient presents a problem that must be solved, whether real or unreal	Assertive behaviour allows to contribute to increase knowledge, lower constraints, and increase patient involvement
Theory of Persuasion Hovland et al. (1953) and Cameron (2009)	Aims to influence model, reinforce or change patient behaviour	Know how to anticipate what the other thinks and says Verbal and non-verbal communication influencing healthy behaviour Opens new paths in perception

(Continued)

Chart 10.1.   (*Continued*)

Theories to Sustain Therapeutic Assertiveness		
Theory and Authors	**Synthesis**	**Behaviours and Attitudes**
 Hall (1980)	Theory Encoding/ Decoding	It is intended that communication is a system of *constant feedback*, in which each participant is simultaneously encoder and decoder with the balance between the message and its meaning	Use of understandable, clear, and positive language, which the other decodes with a hegemonic reading, because it understands
 Bandura (1986)	Social Cognitive Theory	Promoting patient self-efficacy. Teach him how to do it, besides knowing Disengage trust, to get a clear idea of your strengths and how change can be achieved Ensure that the patient knows how to perform a task or action	The professional makes the patient participate and assures in a direct conversation that the patient understands the health instructions, so that the support results in the best way and the patient develops a greater self-care, because it has self-efficacy and assumes the importance of contributing to your health

Source: Own elaboration.

Alberti and Emmons (1973) describe through systematic observations a set of assertive behaviours, whose main components are structured in a non-verbal language (Chart 10.2).

Street and Millay (2001), observing nine videos with patient–doctor inter-actions, developed a coding procedure to evaluate the acts of participation of patients in three categories: (a) when the patient poses questions; (b) when expressing concern; and (c) when it issues assertive responses (p. 63). The authors consider an assertive patient the one who expresses his opinion about health, expresses preferences about treatment, makes recommendations or suggestions, introduces a new topic for the speech, or disagrees with the health professional (p. 64). The results showed that this type of verbal behaviour (asking questions, expressing concern, or having an assertive interaction) represents less than 7% of the total interactions. However, although the number of interactions (9) is not relevant, it was found that patients are more assertive and freer, when profes-sionals have more communication centred on those and that the act of patient participation makes professionals more focused on it (p. 70). Although Street's

Chart 10.2.   Assertive Component in Communication.

---

1. Looking into the eyes, that is, looking directly at the other person with whom you talk, is considered an effective way of declaring that one is sincere about what is said and, in the words, directed
2. The posture of the body, in which the strength of the messages will be increased if one looks forward to the person, stand or sat near him, bow to him, and keep his head right
3. Gestures, in which a message accentuated by appropriate gestures acquires a special emphasis (very exuberant gestures may seem off-purpose)
4. Facial expression, if a person is angry, will not be considered joy
5. The tone of voice, inflection, and volume. For example, a monotonous whisper will hardly convince another person of their seriousness, while a loud voice can prevent communication because it can provoke some resistance in the other person

---

Source: Own elaboration based on Alberti and Emmons (1973).

(1991) study based on the analysis of 41 audiovisual recordings of consultations between professional and patient highlighted that the personal characteristics of patients (such as sex, education and level, and anxiety) as well as communicative styles (questions, opinions, and expressions of concern) influence the *information given* (*information giving*) by the doctor (p. 541).

Parham et al. (2015) investigated the differences in assertiveness related to gender, culture, and ethnicity, and concluded that assertiveness is similar in individuals with the same level and education and *status*. The 231 business students (3 in the USA and 1 in Vietnam) filled Rathus' assertiveness scale. It was also demonstrated that white men were more assertive with African-American women (p. 421).

Patient-focused communication, based on the assertiveness of the health professional, increases patient involvement and confidence and improves outcomes, especially satisfaction (Ahmed & Bates, 2016).

It is therefore necessary to evaluate the qualitative dimension of the information because even if professionals can provide information to answer a patient's question, it can be uninformative if, for example, it is presented in a form of technical jargon that is not understood by the patient (Street, 1991, p. 547).

ACP Model: We Move on to Clarity of Language

The scientific language used in health is not effective (Lalonde, 1981, p. 175) because Science is full of assumptions and questions, as "if", "but" and "perhaps" while messages designed to influence the public must be well heard, clear and unambiguous (p. 175).

It is not by chance that Lalonde (1981) highlights the meaning of the word 'Moi Sui' (sound MOO SUE), which means 'touch, feel, groping' and which reflects, in his opinion (p. 57), a deliberate approach to innovations and creative action, even when safety and scientific predictability are in question.

In the area of health, information must be credible to ensure patient commitment and compliance and credibility will be maximized if the professional is considered a specialist by the patient (Jackson, 1992, p. 201). As a source, the professional uses a language that must be understood by the patient (simple language).

Stableford and Mettger (2007) highlight plain language as a strategic response to the health literacy challenge.

The U.S. Department of Health and Human Services (2000, 2011, 2015) defined plain language or clear language as all oral or written communication that is clear, concise, organized, and does not use technical jargon, with writing, structure, design, and clarity, that allows the reader to easily find, understand, and use this information (Chart 10.3).

Chart 10.3.   Twenty Strategies for Professionals to Communicate More Clearly.

1. *Greet patients warmly*: Welcome everyone with a warm smile, and maintain a friendly attitude throughout the visit
2. *Make real eye contact*: Look into the eyes affable and appropriately throughout the interaction. Consider culture, customs, and beliefs
3. *Make active listening*: Listen carefully, try not to interrupt patients when they speak, pay attention, and answer the questions you ask
4. *Use clear and simple language*: Do not use medical words (technical jargon), or if you use, always explain. Use the words that explain medical information to your friends and family (e.g. stomach or belly instead of abdomen)
5. *Use the patient's words*: The ones that are easily recognized by him. Take note of the words the patient uses to describe his illness, and use them during the conversation
6. *Talk to pauses and moderate the pace of the conversation*: Speak clearly and at a moderate pace (people may have hearing difficulties)
7. *Limit the amount of information, and repeat content*: Prioritize what needs to be discussed, and limit the information to 3–5 key points and re-reinforce the information
8. *Be specific and concrete*: Do not use vague and subjective terms that can be interpreted in different ways
9. *Show graphics*: Draw, use illustrations, or demonstrate, if possible, with templates, tables, drawings, and charts. All images should be simple and designed to demonstrate only important concepts, without detailed anatomy
10. *Demonstrate how it is done, or give concrete examples*: Whether you're exercising or taking medication, demonstrating how to do something can be clearer than a simple verbal explanation
11. *For the final instructions*: Joining text, image, and audio is very positive
12. *Invite the patient to participate*: Encourage patients to ask questions, engage in conversation during visits, and be proactive in their health (empowerment – competence – knowledge – trust)

Chart 10.3. *(Continued)*

---

13. *Encourage questions*: Encourage your patients to ask questions. You can come home now with the written questions, or you can do them in the waiting room
14. *Apply the teach-back method*: Confirm with patients that they understand the information that is passed to them and ask them to repeat in their own words the guidelines they have just received to see if they have understood themselves
15. Review communication strategies with colleagues, with staff during meetings, and ask, for example, a few paths are often born from sharing
16. Advertise through the intranet (alert pop-up), on staff rest room televisions, and in the passage or meeting areas
17. *Pay attention to verbal and non-verbal communication*: In addition to what is said, the posture of the body, the movement of the hands and arms, pauses, and intonation count
18. Observe the patient's posture and listen them, even their short sentences. Make room for the patient to feel at ease
19. Ask open questions too and open the path of empathy as phrases, for example, What can I do for you? What brings you here? How can I help you?
20. In the farewell of the consultation greet again and, if possible, follow the patient's door, reinforce the connection with words of comfort and/ or encouragement

---

Source: Own elaboration based on WHO (2022), CDC (2020), and AHRQ (2016).

Davis and Wolf (2004) report that 75% of the education brochures of the American Physicians Association are written above the average reading level (8th and 9th grades), despite the recognition of the importance of health literacy, this does not happen in practice and the materials are not useful in practice (Davis & Wolf, 2004, p. 596).

Wyer and Shrum (2014) found that visual representations of information can provoke strong emotional reactions, and, if it is easy to recover from memory, can have a greater impact than verbally encoded information (p. 7).

Among other rules that define a clear language, we can observe the following: (1) the use of 'direct' and simple phrases: subject–verb–object, because dense sentences are more difficult for readers than decoding low-frequency words (Schriver et al., 2010, p. 27; Watson, 2019, p. 5); (2) the use of short sentences, because the investigation shows that it is difficult to follow the meaning of the sentence and there is a correlation in the speed of reading and comprehension through the number of words per sentence, the number of prepositions per sentence, and the proportion of unpredictable words. The higher the number, the worse the performance of the readers (Schriver et al., 2010, p. 27); (3) the use of personal pronouns ('Do you/do you want?'); (4) the use of everyday language, avoiding technical jargon or if using it, explain, but paying attention when replacing one word with another so as not to lose the meaning nor the importance, as well as not infantilizing language (Watson, 2019, p. 7); (5) place the main message at the beginning; (6) the use of numbered lists, bullets, and headers to guide people in printed information; (7) the use of tables, graphics, images with subtitles, instead of very extensive texts; (8) leave blank airspaces to allow easier reading; and (9) divides the information into parts and summarizes each 'block', also called 'Chunk and Check'.

So how to communicate clearly? There are already abundant rules about clear language. Credible sources come from international organizations, such as World Health Organization (WHO, 1998, 2013, 2019), CDC (2020), and AHRQ (2016) (Chart 10.3).

Schriver et al. (2010), refer that

> if readers can find the material they need, understand them at the first moment when they read them and use information to perform their task, or the task we want them to perform, it is clear language. (p. 26)

For these authors, the *definition of plain language* cannot be summed up in a set of linguistic techniques (p. 31), such as sentences of 20 words or less, 70% of verbs in active voice, paragraphs up to 10 lines, space in text, or other elements, because here there is still no common definition that can build consensus (Schriver et al., 2010, p. 27).

It is necessary that there *is a standard* (Schriver et al., 2010, p. 31), where there are some techniques that can serve as a *basis for plain language* (Schriver et al., 2010, p. 27).

Regarding the use of 'long sentences', referred to as 'non-promoters of language clarity' (p. 27), Schriver et al. (2010) state that it is not the length of sentences that hinders understanding, but their syntax (rules) and structure (p. 27). They conclude that 'the text improves if the subject is kept close to the predicate' and that the good 'clues' help readers remember the texts (p. 27).

Also, regarding cultural issues, the authors (Schriver et al., 2010, p. 30) consider that research is needed to verify the effectiveness of clear language since not all techniques work in each culture (p. 29).

Watson (2019, p. 6) reinforces this issue by arguing that people may have adequate literacy in their culture, but they may have difficulty in understanding the same concept in another language and other culture.

For the evaluation of these clear language issues, the authors suggest the collection of *qualitative data through focus group* and protocol testing with actual readers and texts and individual interviews, and for the collection of quantitative data suggest control studies (p. 30), through surveys, interviews, or tests with users (p. 31).

Altin and Stock (2016), based on a national cross-sectional telephone survey of German adult patients ($N = 1125$), found that adult Germans with sufficient literacy, whose professionals gave them explanations in a clear and simple way, understood the instructions better, and showed that they were more satisfied with care (p. 1). These patients had score twice as high as expected, as well as those who were involved in the decision had a result four times higher than expected. The study by Altin and Stock (2016) shows the need for organizations to implement more appropriate oral and written communication, involving training the team of healthcare professionals to give them skills to use *already standardized tools*, such as the *teach-back method* (asking the patient to repeat in their own words what they have absorbed) or *chunk & check* (divide the information into small parts, as well as the use of clear language) (p. 7).

Clear language presupposes the use of the active voice and the second person singular (you or you), the limitation of the size of sentences to a maximum of 15 words, the reference of language at the 8th grade level, and the immediate understanding of the contents (Wittenberg et al., 2015).

Among the strategies of verbal and non-verbal communication to communicate clearly, which integrates the very clarity of the relationship, we can highlight the following interventions: greet patients warmly, make eye contact, listen carefully, use the patient's words, decrease the speed of exposure, limit and repeat the content, be specific and concrete, show graphs, demonstrate how it is done, invite patient participation, encourage questions, and *apply teach-back* (Brega et al., 2015, pp. 16–17).

Clear language is a logical and flexible, bilateral response, accessible to the target audience, and is part of the solution to the major health problems (Stableford & Mettger, 2007, pp. 75–76).

ACP Model: Positivity to Give Action and Motivation to Behaviour

Our mind prefers action. Telling someone 'don't do that' can be limiting, and it's preferable to give them an indication of what we'd like them to do and why they should know it. We like to obey better if we understand the importance of our ability. It generates more responsibility. And we're not just talking about managing and educating children. Most human beings prefer to act or do something better, when they understand the importance for themselves, for the group, and for the values they defend.

Neumann et al. (2010), in a research based on non-systematic narrative of literature review (p. 308), conclude that 'positive verbal suggestions of physicians are capable of increasing and/or replacing the effects of medical treatment' (p. 309). These authors reinforce that neurobiological evidence shows that the interaction between the professional and the patient increases the effectiveness of medical treatment (p. 311).

In a systematic review by Di Blasi et al. (2001) and later by Howick et al. (2018) also in a systematic review and meta-analysis where data from studies on empathy interventions (empathy were performed) and interventions with expectations (where professionals sent positive messages to promote patients' positive expectations about outcomes) showed that empathy and positive communication can help improve patient health outcomes.

Chart 10.4. Benefits of Positivity.

Patients	Professionals
Good mental and physical health	Good mental and physical health
Mind change	Mind change
Resilience	Resilience
Placebo effect	Increased positive and constructive
Satisfaction	interaction
Improving health outcomes	Increased satisfaction of teamwork
Decreased pain	Reduction of errors
Blood pressure reduction and other	Satisfaction
physiological issues	Increased efficiency
Medication reduction	Relationship quality
Decreased hospital stay	Better data collection
Reduction of biases	Proper use of time
Improves the quality of decision	Reduction of biases
making	Improves the quality of decision making

Source: Own elaboration based on Berman and Chutka (2016), Enk et al. (2008), Neumann et al. (2010), and Seligman et al. (2005).

Berman and Chutka (2016) and Stewart (1995) reinforce that a positive relationship also contributes to a strengthening of the efficiency and satisfaction of the professional for his profession (p. 243).

Positive language can literally change the brain and assists good mental and physical health. The recommendations consist of avoiding the use of negative words and phrases such as 'I can't', 'never', 'I don't', and 'I won't', and building a framework for ideas through positive phrases, such as 'I choose', 'I can', and 'I'll go' (Corbin et al., 2014). Any negative acts and discourses of the health professional tend to negatively influence the patient (Corbin et al., 2014). Studies by Enk et al. (2008) report that a positive change in expectations, for example, positive verbal cues can lead to reduce pain and improve heart rate, blood pressure, and other physiological measurements.

Negative communication, compared to positive communication, has been associated with a much stronger influence on relational satisfaction (Spitzberg, 2013, p. 94).

Similarly, when the health professional is positive, optimistic, and hopeful, the influence on the patient will have a mirror effect (Corbin et al., 2014). Healthcare providers can urge patient self-efficacy (Bandura, 1977, 1993), using a positive style (Stemple & Hapner, 2014, p. 489).

The construction of knowledge and understanding help to understand why it is important to change (Corbin et al., 2014) so knowing the benefits of healthy lifestyle choices can motivate people to make positive changes (p. 53).

Thomas (1987) suggests that the physician may be the most vital component of the 'placebo effect', through a positive and reinforcing conversation with the patient (p. 1200), confirmed by Wise et al. (2009) in a random test with

601 asthmatics who, with the positive development of expectations, had a better result in symptom reporting and asthma control.

Also in a study by McNeil et al. (1982) on the different ways in which information is presented to patients (the probability of living or the probability of dying), it was evaluated what influence this use of language would have on therapeutic options. 238 outpatients, 424 radiologists, and 491 graduate students who simulated that they had throat cancer were asked, and responses were recorded when patients were presented with options on radiation therapy or surgery. Patients were given two hypotheses to have surgery: (1) to increase the probability of survival; and (2) to reduce the risk of death (p. 1260). The results showed that people more easily selected surgery when they perceived the 'probability of survival', reflecting, here, not only the type of language used but also the positive way to structure the results of the option. Awareness of the effects of presentation can help reduce the biases between professionals and patients and improve the quality of decision making (p. 1262).

For positive psychology, positivity produces a change in the subject's mind, which makes him exchange negative thoughts for positive ones, also altering the goals and limits of his mind (Seligman et al., 2005). The positive subject is characterized by (Luthans et al., 2007, p. 3): (1) having confidence (self-efficacy) to trigger the effort necessary for success in challenging tasks; (2) making a positive attribution (optimism) on present and future success; (3) to persevere towards goals and, when necessary, redirect paths to goals (hope) towards success; and (4) when full of problems and adversities, be resilient.

McCaffrey et al. (2011, p. 121) analyzed an educational and experimental program of positive communication between nurses and internal physicians, demonstrating that this type of communication is associated with increased satisfaction of the teamwork (p. 121), increased patient care (p. 126), and decreased errors.

Stortenbeker et al. (2018) developed a study that quantified the positive communications of general family physicians and evaluated their relationship with patient anxiety. The researchers compared the use of the language of 18 Dutch FGM physicians during 82 consultations in patients with medically unexplained symptoms (SSM) versus patients with clinically explained symptoms (SMS). The content of the message (positive or negative) was differentiated by its frontality (direct or indirect) and related to changes in the patient's state of anxiety (through the STAI Anxiety Traits Inventory). Among the results, 2,590 iterations were identified. For patients with clinically explained symptoms (SM), physicians used more positive and indirect (vs. indirect) negative messages. The anxiety of both patients increased when physicians used more direct (vs. indirect) negative messages. FGM physicians use different types of languages and direct negative messages have been related to increased patient anxiety, so among the study's findings, there is evidence that physicians can better manage patient anxiety by using negative messages indirectly rather than directly.

Diener et al. (1999) reported that happier nations are economically more developed and relatively rich, perhaps because the basic needs and desires of patients are cared for to a greater extent. In a qualitative leap of understanding, health as a state of well-being influences not only the individual in their relationship (e.g. therapeutic relationship), but also the well-being of society that is distinguished by: (1) being a strong rule of law and human rights; (2) where there are low rates of corruption; (3) government is more efficient and effective; (4) taxes on the population are progressive; (5) there are security programs for renting, pensions, unemployment benefits and support for patients, and people with disabilities, in addition to (6) active employment policies, training, employment incentives, and direct job creation; (7) a well-defined field and political freedoms, with property rights, labour, and solid laws and generous unemployment policies, as well as (8) a collection of healthier natural environments, for example, clean air and ample green space.

Seligman et al. of positive psychology (2005) refer that although the causes of a lack of well-being are found in the physical or social environments of poverty, isolation and social exclusion, and stress, individuals can improve their own well-being by practicing appreciation (Seligman et al., 2005), gratitude (Toepfer et al., 2012), and kindness (Lyubomirsky & Layous, 2013). It was also observed that people who act in a happy way tend to make other people happy (Fowler & Christakis, 2008).

Conclusion

Using the ACP Model in an interdependent and aggregated way, consisting of three key communication competencies – assertiveness, clarity, and positivity – transforms the therapeutic relationship. Seeming so simple, it is easy to learn your techniques if the person who wants to learn, knows well the concepts and meanings that are behind these skills. Everything is simple once learned and practices lead to better results. The patient wins and wins the professional, as well as the organization, the communities, and, finally, the society. It seems to be too simple, but the effect of these three aggregate skills has been highlighted by many professionals who have joined the ACP Model in their daily health practices.

The health professionals confirmed the efficacy of the ACP Model in the therapeutic relationship, with the following results: (1) the huge importance they attribute to communication and their communication skills in the context of the therapeutic relationship; (2) the appreciation they give to the use of the competences of assertiveness, clarity of language and positivity, which, even if it may have been overestimated, proved to be a promoter of a motivation and a strong intention of behaviour; and (3) the value they attribute to the application of the aggregated and interdependent ACP Model in their communication performance in the health dyad, allowing the positive results to increase the patient's health literacy, and, therefore, influencing access, understanding, and use of health information and navigate in the health system.

The participants in the FG in this investigation on the communication skills in health and the ACP Model highlight the rational (cognitive) and emotional behaviours, for example, through the use of motivation, controlled and adequate humour provided to the patient (Levinson et al., 2010).

References

Ahmed, R., & Bates, B. R. (2016). To accommodate, or not to accommodate: Exploring patient satisfaction with doctor's accommodative behavior during clinical encounter. *Journal of Communication in HealthCare, 9,*22–32.

AHRQ. (2016). *Health Literacy Universal Precautions Toolkit.* Agency for Healthcare Research and Quality Advancing Excellence in Health Care. www.ahrq.gov

Alberti, R. E., & Emmons, M. L. (2008). *Your perfect right: Assertiveness and equality in your life and relationships.* Impact Publishers.

Alberti, R. E., & Emmons, M. L. (1973). *Comportamento assertivo: Um guia deautoexpressão.* Brasil: InterLivros

Almeida, C. V. (2018). Literacia em saúde: Capacitação dos profissionais de saúde: O lado mais forte da balança. In C. Lopes & C. V. Almeida (Coords.), *Literacia em saúde: Modelos, estratégias e intervenção* (pp. 33–42). Edições ISPA. http://bibliogr afia.bnportugal.gov.pt/bnp/bnp.exe/registo?2016487

Altin, S. V., & Stock, S. S. (2016). The impact of health literacy, patient centered communication and shared decision-making on patients' satisfaction with care received in German primary care practices. *BMC Health Services Research, 16*(450), 1–10.

Bandura, A. (1977). Self-efficacy: Toward a unifying theory of behavior change. *Psychological Review, 84*(2), 191–215.

Bandura, A. (1986). *Social foundations of thought and action: A social cognitive theory.* Prentice-Hall.

Bandura, A. (1993). Perceived self-efficacy in cognitive development and functioning. *Educational Psychologist, 28*(2), 117–148.

Berman, A. C., & Chutka, D. S. (2016). Assessing effective physician-patient communication skills: "Are you listening to me, doc?". *Korean Journal of Medical Education, 28*(2), 243–249.

Brega, A. G., Freedman, M. A. G., LeBlanc, W. G., Barnard, J., Mabachi, N. M., Cifuentes, M., Albright, K., Weiss, B. D., Brach, C., & West, D. R. (2015). Using the health literacy universal precautions toolkit to improve the quality of patient materials. *Journal of Health Communication, 20*(2), 69–76.

Bruning, S. D., & Ledingham, J. A. (1998). Organization-public relationships and consumer satisfaction: The role of relationships in satisfaction mix. *Communication Research Reports, 15*(2), 198–208.

Cameron, K. A. (2009). A practitioner's guide to persuasion: An overview of 15 selected persuasion theories, models and frameworks. *Patient Education & Counseling, 74,* 309–317.

CDC. (2020). What is health literacy?https://www.cdc.gov/healthliteracy/learn/index.html

Cegala, D. J. (2011). An exploration of factors promoting patient participation in primary care medical interviews. *Health Communication, 26,* 427–436.

Coombs, M., & Ersser, S. J. (2004). Medical hegemony in decision-making: A barrier to interdisciplinary working in intensive care? *Journal of Advanced Nursing, 46*(3), 245–252.

Corbin, C. B., McConnell, K. E., Le Masurier, G. C., Corbin, D. E., & Farrar, T. D. (2014). *Health opportunities through physical education.* Human Kinetics.

Davis, T., & Wolf, M. S. (2004). Health literacy: Implications for family medicine. *Family Medicine, 36*(8), 595–598.

Di Blasi, Z., Harkness, E., Ernst, E., Georgiou, A., & Kleijnen, J. (2001). Influence of context effects on health outcomes: A systematic review. *Lancet,357,* 757–762.

Diener, E., Suh, E. M., Lucas, R. E., & Smith, H. L. (1999). Subjective well-being: Three decades of progress. *Psychological Bulletin, 125*(2), 276–302.

Enk, P., Benedetti, F., & Schedlowski, M. (2008). New insights into placebo and nocebo responses. *Neuron, 59,* 195–206.

Espanha, R., & Ávila, P. (2016). Health literacy survey Portugal: A contribution for the knowledge on health and communications. *Procedia Computer Science, 100*, 1033–1041. https://10.1016/j.procs.2016.09.277

Fowler, J. H., & Christakis, N. A. (2008). Dynamic spread of happiness in a large social network: Longitudinal analysis over 20 years in the Framingham Heart Study. *BMJ, 337*. https://doi.org/10.1136/bmj.a2338

Hall, S. (1980). Encoding/decoding. In S. Hall, D. Hobson, A. Lowe & P. Willis (Eds.), *Culture, media, language: Working papers in cultural studies* (pp. 128–138). London: Hutchinson.

Hovland, C., Janis, I., & Kelley, H. (1953). *Communication and persuasion*. Yale University Press.

Howick, J., Moscrop, A., Mebius, A., Fanshawe, T. R., Lewith, G., Bishop, F. L., Mistiaen, P., Roberts, N. W., Dieninytė, E., Hu, X. Y., Aveyard, P., & Onakpoya, I. J. (2018). Effects of empathic and positive communication in healthcare consultations: A systematic review and meta-analysis. *Journal of the Royal Society of Medicine, 111*(7), 240–252. https://doi.org/10.1177/0141076818769477

Jackson, L. D. (1992). Information complexity and medical communication: The effects of technical language and amount of information in a medical message. *Health Communication, 4*(3), 197–210.

Kim, J. N., & Grunig, J. E. (2011). Problem solving and communicative action: A situational theory of problem solving. *Journal of Communication, 61*, 120–149.

Koh, H. K., Brach, C., Harris, L. M., & Parchman, M. L. (2013). A proposed 'health literate care model' would constitute a systems approach to improving patients' engagement in care. *Health Affairs (Millwood), 32*(2), 357–367. https://doi.org/10.1377/hlthaff.2012.1205

Lalonde, M. (1981). *A new perspective on the health of Canadians*. Information Canada.

Levinson, W., Lesser, C. S, & Epstein, R. M. (2010). Developing physician communication skills for patients-centered care. *Health Affairs, 29*(7), 1310–1318. https://doi.org/10.1377/hlthaff.2009.0450

Luthans, F., Youssef, C. M., & Avolio, B. J. (2007). *Psychological capital: Developing the human competitive edge*. Oxford: Oxford University Press.

Lyubomirsky, S., & Layous, K. (2013). How do simple positive activities increase well-being? *Current Directions in Psychological Science, 22*(1), 57–62.

McCaffrey, R. G., Hayes, R., Stuart, W., Cassel, A., Farrell, C., Miller-Reyes, S., & Donaldson, A. (2011). An educational program to promote positive communication and collaboration between nurses and medical staff. *Journal for Nurses in Staff Development: Official Journal of the National Nursing Staff Development Organization, 27*(3), 121–127. https://doi.org/10.1097/NND.0b013e318217b3ce

McNeil, B. J., Pauker, S. G., Sox, H. C., & Tversky, A. (1982). On the elicitation of preferences for alternative therapies. *New England Journal of Medicine, 306*(21), 1259–1262.

Miller, T. (2016). Health literacy and adherence to medical treatment in chronic and acute illness: A meta-analysis. *Patient Education & Counseling, 99*, 1079–1086.

Morris, M. W., & Keltner, D. (2000). How emotions work: The social functions of emotional expression in negotiations. *Research in Organizational Behavior, 22*, 1–50.

Neumann, M., Eldelhauser, F., Kreps, G. L., Scheffer, C., Lutz, G., Tauschel, D., & Visser, A. (2010). Can patient–provider interaction increase the effectiveness of medical treatment or even substitute it? An exploration on why and how to study the specific effect of the provider. *Patient Education & Counseling, 80*, 307–314.

Parham, J. B., Lewis, C. C., Fretwell, C. E., Irwin, J. G., & Schrimsher, M. R. (2015). Influences on assertiveness: Gender, national culture, and ethnicity. *Journal of Management Development, 34*(4), 421–439.

Sabia, S., Guéguen, A., Marmot, M. G., Shipley, M. J., Ankri, J., & Singh-Manoux, A. (2010). Does cognition predict mortality in midlife? Results from the Whitehall II cohort study. *Neurobiology Aging, 31*(4), 688–695. https://doi.org/10.1016/j.neurobiolaging.2008.05.007

Schriver, K., Cheek, A. L., & Mercer, M. (2010). The research basis of plain language techniques: Implications for establishing standards. *Clarity*, 26–33. https://www.researchgate.net/publication/285927928_The_research_basis_of_plain_language_techniques_Implications_for_establishing_standards

Seligman, M. E., Steen, T. A., Park, N., & Peterson, C. (2005). Positive psychology progress: Empirical validation of interventions. *American Psychologist, 60*(5), 410–421.

Sørensen, K., Van den Broucke, S., Fullam, J., Doyle, G., Pelikan, J., Slonska, Z., & Brand, H. (2012). Health literacy and public health: A systematic review and integration of definitions and models. *BMC Public Health, 12,* 80.

Spitzberg, B. H. (2013). (Re)Introducing communication competence to the health professions. *Journal of Public Health Research, 2*(3), 126–135.

Stableford, S., & Mettger, W. (2007). Plain language: A strategic response to the health literacy challenge. *Journal of Public Health Policy, 28*(1), 71–93. https://doi.org/10.1057/palgrave.jphp.3200102

Stein, S., & Book, H. (2006). *The EQ edge: Emotional intelligence and your success.* Jossey-Bass.

Stemple, J. C., & Hapner, E. R. (2014). *Voice therapy: Clinical case studies.* Plural.

Stewart, M. A. (1995). Effective physician-patient communication and health outcomes: A review. *CMAJ, 152,* 1423–1433.

Stortenbeker, I. A., Houwen, J., Lucassen, P. L., Stappers, H. W., Assendelft, W. J., van Dulmen, S., Hartman, T. C., & Das, E. (2018). Quantifying positive communication: Doctor's language and patient anxiety in primary care consultations. *Patient Education & Counseling, 101,* 1577–1584.

Street, R. L. (1991). Information-giving in medical consultation. The influence of patient's communicative styles and personal characteristics. *Social Science & Medicine, 32*(5), 541–548.

Street, R. L., & Millay, B. (2001). Analyzing patient participation. *Health Communication, 13*(1), 61–73.

Thomas, K. (1987). General practice consultations: Is there any point in being positive? *British Medical Journal, 294,* 1200–1202.

Toepfer, S. M., Cichy, K., & Peters, P. (2012). Letters of gratitude: Further evidence for author benefits. *Journal Happiness Studies, 13*(1), 187–201.

U.S. Department of Health and Human Services. (2000). *Healthy People 2010.* U.S. Government Printing Office.

U.S. Department of Health and Human Services. (2011). *National action plan to improve health literacy.* U.S. Department of Health and Human Services.

U.S. Department of Health and Human Services. (2015). *Health literacy online: A guide to simplifying the user experience.* Office of Disease Prevention and Health Promotion. https://health.gov/healthliteracyonline/

Vaz de Almeida, C. (2020). O contributo das competências de comunicação dos médicos e enfermeiros para a literacia em saúde: O Modelo ACP Assertividade (A), Clareza (C) E Positividade (P) Na Relação Terapêutica. Zenodo. https://zenodo.org/badge/DOI/10.5281/zenodo.4495585.svg; https://doi.org/10.5281/zenodo.4495585

Vaz de Almeida, C. (2022). ACP Model – Assertiveness, clarity and positivity: A communication and health literacy model for health professionals. In C. Vaz de Almeida & S. Ramos (Eds.), *Handbook of research on assertiveness, clarity, and positivity in health literacy.* IGI Books. https://www.igi-global.com/book/assertiveness-clarity-positivity-health-literacy/273602; https://doi.org/doi:10.4018/978-1-7998-8824-6.ch 001. ISBN13: 9781799888246|ISBN10: 179988824X|EISBN13: 9781799888253

Vaz de Almeida, C., & Belim, C. (2021). Health professionals' communication competences as a light on the patient pathway: The Assertiveness, Clarity, and Positivity (ACP) Model.

International Journal of Applied Research on Public Health Management, 6(1), 14–29. https://www.igi-global.com/article/health-professionals-communication-competences-as-a-light-on-the-patient-pathway/267793; https://doi.org/10.4018/IJARPHM.2021010102

Watson, J. C. (2019). Talking the talk: Enhancing clinical ethics with health literacy best practices. *HEC Forum*, 1–23.

WHO. (2013). *Health literacy: The solid facts*. OMS.

WHO. (2019). Improving health through health literacy. *Panorama*, 5(2–3), 123–329.

WHO. (2022). *WHO principles for effective communications*. https://www.who.int/about/communications/principles

Wise, M., & Nutbeam, D. (2007). Enabling health systems transformation: what progress has been made in re-orienting health services? *Promotion & Education, 2*, 23–27.

Wittenberg, E., Goldsmith, J., Ferrel, B., & Platt. C. S. (2015). Enhancing communication related to symptom management through plain language. *Journal of Pain and Symptom Management, 50*(5), 707–711.

World Health Organization (WHO). (1998). *Health promotion glossary*. WHO.

Wyer, R. S., & Shrum, L. J. (2014). The role of comprehension processes in communication and persuasion. *Media Psychology*, 1–33.

Chapter 11

Patient Safety Education and Digital Technology Contributions

Ana Marinho Diniz[a], Susana Ramos[a], Karina Pecora[b] and José Branco[b]

[a]Centro Hospitalar Universitário de Lisboa Central, Lisboa, Portugal
[b]Brazilian Patient Safety Institute, São Paulo, Brasil

Abstract

Adverse events in health care became more evident at the beginning of the 21st century, being an emerging problem worldwide and impacting the lives of people receiving health care, contributing to preventable injuries and deaths. This evidence has motivated the development of specific training in the area of patient safety with a strong focus on the education and training of health professionals, and, more recently, it also aimed at patient, informal caregiver and all citizens. In this sense, the use of digital technology for patient safety training has been an important challenge and proves to be a good solution for training and continuous learning, both for professionals and people in general. The use of multimedia, videos, games, simulators, among others, are effectively essential resources to improve people's health literacy and safety of care.

This chapter presents a narrative review on patient safety training and the contributions of digital technology. The experience report will also be used, presenting some examples of quality improvement projects developed by Portuguese and Brazilian entities, in training contexts, highlighting the importance of investing in the health literacy of professionals, patients/informal caregivers and civil society, through applying specific techniques and using digital technology.

Keywords: Digital technology; health literacy; patient safety; quality improvement projects; training and education; health education

Technology-Enhanced Healthcare Education:
Transformative Learning for Patient-Centric Health, 145–164
Copyright © 2024 by Ana Marinho Diniz, Susana Ramos, Karina Pecora and José Branco
Published under exclusive licence by Emerald Publishing Limited
doi:10.1108/978-1-83753-598-920231011

Introduction

Global health policies have evolved to promote the population's right to health protection. They also aim to ensure equity in the access to decent, timely and appropriate health care for the person's particular situation in case of illness, according to the best available scientific evidence, respecting the good practices of quality and safety in health (Portugal, 2022; WHO, 2020, 2021). However, annually millions of people are harmed or die due to unsafe healthcare worldwide. The evolution of knowledge in this area has allowed for the recognition that patient safety incidents are reality in today's healthcare systems. In 2019, in a resolution of the World Health Organization (WHO) General Assembly, patient safety was considered one of the priorities of global health (WHO, 2021).

Several countries have developed studies to estimate the rate of adverse events associated with health care, characterizing their nature, and assessing their impact and avoidability (Sousa et al., 2018). The hospital context is one of the most frequent fields of investigation. However, factors, such as the increase in the population's average life expectancy, the chronicity of diseases, and the complexity of clinical situations, have increased the variability of care settings, extrapolating the boundaries of these organizations (Vincent & Amalberti, 2015).

The education and training of health professionals, patients themselves and their informal caregivers are essential tools in the process of empowering them to recognize the existence of risks associated with the particularities of the different care environments and practices (Almeida, 2020). In the context of education and training, solutions and strategies may be found to promote risk reduction and control, thus preventing possible errors and increasing care safety (Stevenson et al., 2012).

In 2009, the WHO, aware of the issue and the need to change the safety culture in health organizations, published the Curriculum Guide for Patient Safety, proposing the integration of 11 areas in the training programs of health organizations (WHO, 2011). Increasingly, it has also been important to increase citizen literacy in the area of care safety, and the WHO proposed the 'Patient for Patient Safety' challenge. This movement aimed to draw attention to the need to promote the education and training of patients and their caregivers. By promoting the involvement, empowerment and capacity building of citizens for active participation in health care, they can certainly contribute to their safety. In this line of thought, the patient is no longer a simple care receiver, and can contribute to safer care (Ramos, 2020).

The 'Speak UP' program developed by the Joint Commission in 2002 is an excellent example of a strategy to promote citizen literacy in healthcare safety, with the advantage of being replicable in different contexts and realities. This program provides, in digital support, several checklists, booklets and educational videos, which aim to contribute to the empowerment and capacity building of citizens, taking an active role in the promotion of healthcare safety (Ramos & Almeida, 2020).

The development of the digital age and digital transformation has imposed a huge challenge to health organizations, making it essential to develop health ecosystems that empower people to have a greater participation in managing their health and promoting well-being, previously supported by health teams (Magalhães, 2021). In addition to this emerging and global need, the digital and technological evolution has also brought about the possibility of using new strategies and modalities for the training and education of professionals, as well as people in general in the area of patient safety.

Patient Safety Training and the Challenge of Using Digital Technology

The promotion of patient safety requires a continuous, concerted and global action of organizations and health systems, integrating all their stakeholders. This premise is reflected in the WHO Global Plan of Action for Patient Safety 2021–2030, which establishes seven strategic objectives in order to prevent harm and avoid the deaths of millions of people as a result of unsafe health care (WHO, 2021) (Fig. 11.1). Of these, we highlight objectives 4 and 5, which set goals for the involvement of patients and families, as well as for the promotion of health professionals' training in patient safety, respectively.

Among the initiatives to improve the education of health professionals, we highlight the Patient Safety Curriculum Guide (WHO, 2011), which was initially aimed at physicians, but was later presented in a multiprofessional version. This guide emerges with the proposal of 11 themes in the area of patient safety, reinforcing the importance of their inclusion in the curricular subjects of educational institutions and the training programs of health organizations (Fig. 11.2). The

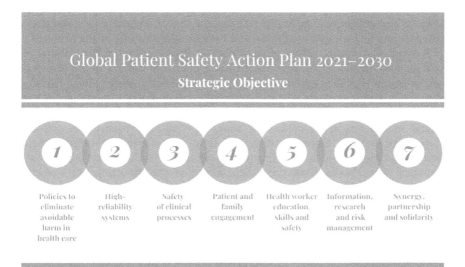

Fig. 11.1. Strategic Goals of the WHO Global Patient Safety Action Plan 2021–2030. *Source*: Own elaboration based on WHO (2021).

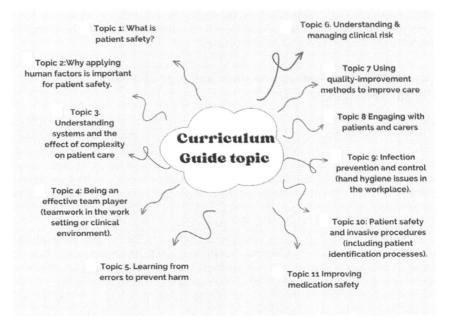

Topic 1: What is patient safety?

Topic 2:Why applying human factors is important for patient safety.

Topic 3. Understanding systems and the effect of complexity on patient care

Topic 4: Being an effective team player (teamwork in the work setting or clinical environment).

Topic 5. Learning from errors to prevent harm

Topic 6. Understanding & managing clinical risk

Topic 7 Using quality-improvement methods to improve care

Topic 8 Engaging with patients and carers

Topic 9: Infection prevention and control (hand hygiene issues in the workplace).

Topic 10: Patient safety and invasive procedures (including patient identification processes).

Topic 11 Improving medication safety

Curriculum Guide topic

Fig. 11.2.   Topics to be Included in Patient Safety Education and Training Programs. *Source*: Own elaboration based on WHO (2011).

designed contents have as pedagogical principles to contextualize the concepts in patient safety and use real examples for a better understanding of the problem.

A practical example, with a great impact on patient safety, is the training on 'safe patient identification'. Identification is a basic assumption in the care process to ensure that the right care is provided to the right person. It is therefore essential that professionals and patients/caregivers understand and take ownership of good practices to increase patient safety throughout the patient journey. Digital technology, in the context of training, in the classroom or virtually, is an excellent resource, through strategies such as videos with real testimonies, of patients and professionals, reporting identification errors. Educational games and simulated cases also facilitate the understanding of the importance of a correct patient identification in the various stages of the patient's journey and the good practices to be systematically adopted by all participants (Fig. 11.3).

Understanding risks, knowing how to recognize and manage them, being able to apply strategies of detection, reporting and analysis of events are contents that integrate the curriculum guide. It also proposes a systemic vision of the process, placing patient safety as an inseparable part of teamwork, clear and concise communication at all strategic levels. The way we establish communication with patients and among multidisciplinary teams complements the strategies to establish and sustain a culture of patient safety in health organizations (WHO, 2011).

Patient safety education in health professions schools (medicine, nursing, pharmacy, among others) is scarce or non-existent. On the other hand, in hospitals

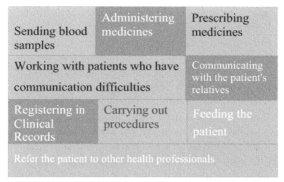

Fig. 11.3.   Examples of 'Moments' for Correct Patient Identification. *Source*: Own elaboration based on the WHO (2011).

and other healthcare organizations in addition to the lack of basic knowledge and skills, the culture and working environment are against many of the requirements for safe practice (Wu & Busch, 2019).

The multiprofessional approach of the WHO Guide, also reflects the need for a global and integrated approach, involving all health professionals and students in patient safety issues, in order to turn patient safety incidents into rare events (Leotsakos et al., 2014). The 'Global Action Plan for Patient Safety 2021–2030: Towards Eliminating Avoidable Harm in Healthcare' aims to 'achieve the maximum possible reduction of avoidable harm due to unsafe healthcare worldwide'. To this end, it proposes, among its strategic objectives, an emphasis on education, skills and health worker safety, which makes the need to invest in the training of professionals in patient safety (WHO, 2021).

Training and simulation in the area of patient safety are therefore a priority in health care, contributing to the prevention of adverse events and increasing healthcare safety. In highly complex contexts and environments, such as operating rooms, intensive care, emergency services, delivery rooms and other health areas, the use of case simulation and the use of digital technology are an excellent teaching and training methods for health professionals, particularly in the development of technical skills (e.g. device handling) and non-technical skills (e.g. communication and teamwork) (Garcia et al., 2021). Failures in communication and teamwork are contributing factors to adverse events, which are often identified in studies, in processes of root cause(s) analysis of adverse events or in complaints (Costar & Hall, 2020; Weaver et al., 2014). Several organizations have developed support programs and tools (e.g. checklists, briefings and handoffs) to improve the teamwork and team performance (Costar & Hall, 2020).

A systematic literature review conducted by Weaver et al. (2014) showed that team training can have a moderate- to high-quality impact on the care processes and patient outcomes, both in terms of reduced morbidity and mortality and reduced occurrence of adverse events (Weaver et al., 2014). The pedagogical methods identified in the analyzed articles refer to methods based on information (e.g. classroom), demonstration (e.g. videos and behavioural models) and practice (e.g. simulation and role-playing). They were applied in settings such as intensive care, surgery and emergency care.

In Portugal and Brazil, an example to be highlighted within the scope of training in patient safety for health professionals is the International Course in Quality in Health and Patient Safety, resulting from a partnership between the National School of Public Health Sérgio Arouca of the Oswaldo Cruz Foundation (Brazil) and the National School of Public Health of the New University of Lisbon (Portugal). This distance learning course uses digital technologies, based on four fundamental pillars: pedagogical material available online, virtual learning environment, tutoring system and academic–pedagogical follow-up. It is a university extension course that contains several pedagogical tools available to students and, at the same time, provides tutoring with teachers and experts in the field of patient safety. Virtual tutorial sessions and videoconferences are also held with national and international experts promoting reflection in practice and discussion about issues related to patient safety (Reis et al., 2021).

In Portugal, regarding the training and empowerment of the citizen in the area of patient safety, several initiatives have emerged, particularly the several online courses for the citizen promoted by the Directorate-General of Health, which aim to increase the citizen's literacy in this area (Portugal, 2019). This initiative arises under the Priority Areas defined for the Pilot Project 'Health Care Safety Literacy' in 2017 and covers six themes of patient safety (Fig. 11.4) (Portugal, 2017). These projects have leveraged national and local dynamics in different health organizations, driving the integration of the topic into the agenda of politicians, health professionals, patients and citizens in Portugal.

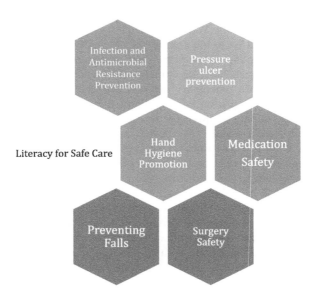

Fig. 11.4.   Priority Areas of the 'Healthcare Safety Literacy' Pilot Project. *Source*: Own elaboration based on the pilot project 'Health Care Safety Literacy' (Portugal, 2017).

Experience in Portugal

The Centro Hospitalar Universitário Lisboa Central (CHULC) is a nationally and internationally certified and accredited health organization, with around 8,000 professionals, which is part of the Portuguese National Health System. It is made up of six hospital units, which bring together a history of more than five centuries, and since then it has occupied a central position in clinical teaching in Portugal (http://www.chlc.min-saude.pt/patrimonio-cultural/nota-historica/).

In support of the exponential development and technological innovation of clinical procedures, this hospital centre has more than two decades of work developed in the area of Quality and Patient Safety. Its strategy for Patient Safety aims to promote the detection, prevention and control of risk factors, as a way of contributing to the development of safer working systems and practices. In this sense, the Patient Safety Office (PSO) was created, which is a support structure of the Board of Directors, which integrates its Quality and Safety System, participating in the Quality and Safety Commission of this health organization.

This office's area of action is based on the pursuit of the various challenges of the WHO and the National Plans for Patient Safety of the Directorate-General for Health, contributing to the development of an organizational culture of safety. Aware of the importance of professionals recognizing that risks can be reduced and controlled, assuming the values that guide safe practices in the area of risk management and patient safety (WHO, 2011), it has developed work and training in various dimensions, namely:

- Safety Culture Environment
- Health and Safety Communication
- Surgical Safety
- Safety Medication
- Corret Patient Identification
- Patient Falls and Pressure Ulcers
- Prevention Healthcare Associated Infections
- Incident Reporting System and Adverse Events Root Cause Analysis
- Safety Management in the *Delirium* Patient
- Avoiding Catheter and Tubing Mis-Connections
- Good Practices for Safe Care – Patient Safety Projects
- Challenges for Leadership and Governance in Promoting Safe Care
- Promoting Child Safety
- Health Literacy for Safe Care
- Patient Safety Research
- Safety in Telehealth

The development of multidisciplinary training activities, within the scope of the admission and integration programs of the institution or in the continuous training of professionals, has become one of the main activities developed annually by the PSO, focusing on central themes of Risk Management and Patient Safety, presented in Table 11.1.

On-the-job training has also been one of the strategies used, in order to promote the training of professionals in the area of patient safety. In these sessions, promoted by the PSO and local interlocutors, incidents, near-events, alerts and publications (articles, clinical guidelines/standards, internal policies and procedures) are disseminated, to encourage the teams' critical analysis and the promotion of safe practices in their respective contexts.

In 2019, the training activities promoted and streamlined internally by the PSO were conducted in person, in a total of 468 hours and reached a total of 2,257 trainees. In 2020, the training activities carried out, had a total of 1,119 participants. It should be noted the need, in that year, to restructure the training activity given the context imposed by the pandemic by COVID-19. The option for digital methodologies proved to be an alternative and effective strategy, translated into a high adherence in participation. This type of strategy also facilitated the participation of external trainers, national and international, as it did not require travel, increasing the diversity of perspectives and sharing.

In 2021, it was possible to resume face-to-face activities. However, the option to maintain the digital strategies was inevitable for the following years. When comparing the face-to-face methodology with the digital one, the differences

Table 11.1.   Patient Safety Training at the CHULC.

Main Themes

* Patient Safety and Risk Management
* Notification and Management Incident
* Root Cause Analysis of Patient Safety Incidents
* Managing Safety in the Medication Circuit
* Safety in the Preparation and Administration of Medicines
* Safety in the Use of Totally Implantable Central Venous Catheters
* Safety in the Use of Medicines in Pediatrics
* Safe Prescribing of Medicines
* Safety Patient Identification
* Safe Transmission of Information in Care Transitions
* Prevention and Management of Falls in Hospitals
* Safety Management in the Delirium Patient
* Safe Care for Women and Newborns
* Child Safety
* Safer professionals, safer patients
* Patient Safety: From Theory to Clinical Practice. Ongoing Projects at the CHULC

Source: Elaborated by the author.

become evident, with regard to the number of trainees covered, number of training hours and volume of training achieved, as expressed in Table 11.2.

The methodologies transversally used in the training activities are:

- Presentation of good practices recommended by national and international reference entities, with the participation of internal or external national and international experts.
- Dissemination of research studies, with evidence of results for patient safety, with particular emphasis on the work developed in the institution.
- Reflection on professional practices through the analysis of scientific articles and real case studies presented in training videos, preferably using situations that have occurred in the organization and reported in the internal patient safety incident reporting system.
- Simulation of cases and training in the use of specific methodologies of risk management and incident analysis, namely of instruments available in the organization.
- Analysis and discussion of patient safety alerts or other informative materials (e.g. videos, posters and infographics with safety recommendations) shared across the organization as a response to cross-cutting issues identified (e.g. LASA Medicines – Look Alike, Sound Alike).
- Sharing of experiences with testimonies of patients, relatives, informal caregivers and professionals involved in adverse events or who have lived healthcare experiences in improvement processes under development in the institution. In this case, the most frequently used strategy is to show videos with testimonies or to share them in real-time through videoconferences.
- Sharing of experiences of quality improvement and patient safety projects, promoted by local interlocutors in their respective work contexts, with the support and guidance of the PSO, using the PDSA (Plan, Do, Check and Act) methodology, as a response to problems identified in the risk assessment processes carried out annually or in the analysis of incidents, including near-events that occurred in the services. The central themes of the projects currently in progress at the CHULC are presented in Table 11.3.

Table 11.2. Volume of Patient Safety Training Conducted at the CHULC – 2021 and 2022.

Modality	Presencial		Digital	
Year	2021	2022	2021	2022
No. hours training	43	114	26	32
No. trainees	440	1,125	1,433	1,597
Volume of training	1,626	2,464	2,568	3,168

Source: Elaborated by the author.

Table 11.3.   Examples of Quality Improvement and Patient Safety Projects Underway at the CHULC.

Issue	Methodologies
'Right care for the right patient' – Unequivocal identification of patients	• Questionnaire for professionals • Observation of identification practices at different moments (admission, preparation and administration of medicines, application of blood and haemoderivative transfusion, collection of biological products, performance of complementary diagnostic and therapeutic examinations, and transfer of care and discharge of the patient) before and after intervention in the team
Communication and transmission of information for continuity of care	• Observation of practices (analysis of the duration and quality of information transmitted during transitions of care) – Visit to units that have implemented ISBAR – Questionnaire for professionals
Safety in the use of the medicine	• Analysis of incidents and near misses reported in the unit – Questionnaire for professionals – Observation of medicine preparation and administration practices • Implementation of independent double-checking in the preparation and administration of medicines, with a recording of errors detected by the second professional in the check (identify the most frequent causes)
Falls risk in patients with severe thrombocytopenia or on oral anticoagulation	• Multi-incident analysis – Post-fall protocol
'Phlebitis associated with peripheral venous catheterization and the use of intravenous drugs/ fluids'	Research project that counted with the participation of a postgraduate student from the Portuguese Catholic University in training at the PSO, and with the Intravascular Devices Working Group of the CHULC's Medical Area. • Integrative literature review – Multi-incident analysis – Questionnaire applied to professionals – Observation of practices in the preparation and administration of medicines
Falls risk associated with the use of medicines	Research project with the participation of a postgraduate student from the National School of Public Health at the New University of Lisbon in training at the PSO. • Integrative literature review – Multi-incident analysis

Table 11.3.   *(Continued)*

Issue	Methodologies
Infection prevention and control practices in the preparation and administration of medicines IV	Research project with the participation of two postgraduate students from the Nursing School of Lisbon and the Portuguese Catholic University, in training at the PSO • *Scoping* review – Observation of practices in the preparation and administration of medicines IV
Prevention of mechanical restraint in the elderly in hospital settings	Research project with the participation of a postgraduate student from the Lisbon School of Nursing on placement at the PSO – Integrative literature review • Observation of the practices of health professionals in relation to mechanical restraint in the provision of care to the elderly – Application of questionnaire to health professionals – Conducting structured interviews with family members/informal caregivers of hospitalized older people
Telehealth and therapeutic reconciliation on patient admission	Research project developed by a member of the PSO team attending the International Course on Quality and Patient Safety at the National School of Public Health and with the participation of a postgraduate student from the Portuguese Catholic University, in training at the PSO • Observational, quantitative study

Source: Elaborated by the author.

As a result of the global analysis of the incidents, the PSO initiated a new approach, proactive and promoting the safety culture in the organization. Thus, on 18 June 2021, a weekly item was created in the internal newsletter of the CHULC, called 'Patient Safety: from theory to practice', which is sent by email to all professionals of the institution. It addresses various topics, in a summarized way, but focused on the practical application of safety recommendations, referring to bibliography that can be consulted if the professional is interested in the topic. It also counts on the participation of local interlocutors, experts in the areas in question, in the preparation or review of the contents. In this way, it is intended to awaken professionals to current relevant topics, guiding them towards good practices and involving them in the process of changing the organizational safety culture (Table 11.4).

The importance of patient, family and informal caregivers' involvement and empowerment for the safety of the care provided has also been one of the targets of this team's work. Under the pilot project 'Health Care Safety Literacy' (Portugal, 2017) coordinated by the Directorate-General for Health and initiated

Table 11.4.   Patient Safety Topics Published at the CHULC.

'Patient Safety: From Theory to Practice': Subjects Publish Weekly in the Institutional Newsletter	
• Adverse drug reactions	Management of the patient's own medication
• Patient identification	Empowering the adult patient and caregiver to return home safely
• LGBTQIA+ patient safety	Exposure to cancer patient 'excreta'
• Safe connections	Zero tolerance for female genital mutilation
• Alternative strategies to mechanical restraint in the elderly	Right care for the right patient
• Risk of falling associated with the use of medicines	Abbreviations, Acronyms and Symbols: What do they mean for patient (in)safety?
• Phlebitis associated with peripheral venous catheters	Mechanical restraint and patient safety
• Surgical fire	Safe maintenance of fully implanted intravascular devices
• Patient involvement in patient safety	Safety in women's health
• Suicide prevention	Medication reconciliation
• Food allergy	Patient Safety Training and Simulation: a priority for safe care
• Patient safety in the transition of care	Incident Reporting System: a tool for patient safety
• Patient safety in palliative care	Management of the physical environment in fall prevention
• Safety of the elderly	Drug allergies
• Green Operating Theatre – Environmental Sustainability	Clinical supervision of students and the safety of care
• Safety in surgical positioning	Patient safety research
• Adherence to medication regime	Health literacy, sustainability, tobacco and patient safety
• *Burnout* and patient safety	Health literacy – a contribution to surgical site infection prevention
• Information transfer in the transition – ISBAAR	In the vortex of Digital Transformation in Healthcare
• Mental health promotion in the peripartum period	Safe transportation of children
• Patient safety in the use of off-label medicines	Active Ageing and Safety in Medicines Management
• Playing safely in hospital	The 12 right ones in preparing and administering medicines
• Human rights and patient safety	Preventing errors in vaccine use
• Alarm fatigue	Telehealth and patient safety

Source: Elaborated by the author.

in 2018 at the CHULC, training sessions were developed aimed at citizens and professionals. They addressed topics related to six areas defined as priorities for Portugal, with the involvement of the Arroios Parish Council, the Order of Pharmacists and the Portuguese Operating Rooms Nurses Association and other CHULC structures. Thus, the sessions focused on:

- Hand hygiene
- Safe medication use
- Surgical safety
- Infections and antibiotics resistances prevention
- Preventing pressure ulcers
- Falls prevention

This approach to patient safety topics within civil society had already been initiated by the PSO in 2013, when it began its annual patient safety campaigns (Diniz et al., 2022). These initiatives, inspired by the 'Patient for patient safety' movement, have focused on different topics over the years, as shown in Fig. 11.5.

These campaigns, aimed at health professionals, patients, relatives, informal carers and civil society, include several initiatives:

- Lecture cycles, both face-to-face and online, open to the public, with the participation of experts and testimonials from patients and carers.
- Preparation and dissemination of information materials in digital and physical support (e.g. posters, flyers, educational games, videos aimed at professionals and citizens).
- Articulation with Professional Orders and Associations, Leagues and Patients Associations and Volunteers.

The need for greater patient involvement was also observed in the request made by some CHULC units to the PSO for the development of projects and activities aimed at their users/informal caregivers, with the collaboration of local interlocutors. An example of this is the participation in sessions aimed at informal caregivers on 'Patient safety on returning home', within the scope of the project organized by the Group for the support of informal caregivers of the

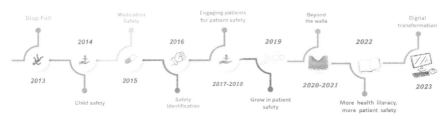

Fig. 11.5.   Patient Safety Campaigns – CHULC. *Source*: Elaborated by the author.

haemato-oncological patient or in sessions aimed at patients being treated at the haemato-oncology day hospital on safe identification (Diniz et al. (2022).

Brazilian Experience

In line with the international patient safety movement since the publication of the book report 'To Err is Human' (1999) by the Institute of Medicine, the Brazilian Institute for Patient Safety (IBSP) was created in 2001 to provide and disseminate relevant educational content on Quality of Care and Safety to health professionals and institutions in our country.

IBSP believes that this transformation is highly dependent on the need for healthcare organizations to place 'Quality and Safety' as a first priority among institutional strategies aimed at reducing harm by implementing educational initiatives focused on improving care processes. Avoiding, preventing, improving adverse outcomes and providing quality through risk management and waste reduction becomes imperative for health care.

Among our various educational actions, we bring methodology and tools to promote critical thinking and systemic vision in quality and safety. Our approach promotes a three-dimensional look focused on process analysis, technical scientific knowledge and support for decision making regarding a process or line of care.

In this sense, and in partnership with health stakeholders and the scientific committee of the IBSP, we developed an educational initiative called 'Validation of Good Safety Practices' based on a critical and qualitative approach to the care process through the analysis of the reliability of barriers, promoting the adequacy of results, reduction of incidents and problems related to patient safety. The chosen theme was the prevention of venous thromboembolism (VTE), a potentially lethal and highly preventable condition. Despite the implementation of the VTE protocol being a recommendation widely disseminated by the medical literature for over 30 years, the average adequacy of prophylaxis in hospitals is 50% (Curtarelli et al., 2019).

VTE is the leading preventable cause of death in hospitalized patients. The pharmacological methods currently available for prevention are safe, effective, cost-effective and supported by several official guidelines, but many scientific publications continue to show that these preventive methods are significantly underused (Maynard, 2016). These data corroborate the need to improve patient safety regarding VTE prevention through institutional policies.

The IBSP strategy for this project was to choose a worldwide reference recommendation in order to officially establish improvement strategies to support health institutions and professionals in decision making related to VTE prophylaxis adequacy initiatives. Our choice was to incorporate the recommendations of the Agency for Healthcare Research and Quality (AHRQ), the main American Federal Agency in charge of improving the safety and quality of the healthcare system in the USA.

Published in 2008, the guide 'Preventing Hospital-Acquired Venous Thromboembolism: A Guide for Effective Quality Improvement' addresses quality improvement initiatives carried out in large hospital centres in the USA, in order to corroborate with leaders and professionals in the search for improvements to prevent one of the most important problems faced by hospitalized patients, in-hospital VTE.

In accordance with the AHRQ recommendations, the project was structured around three pillars, among them, multidisciplinary education aimed at filling the gap of difficulty in implementing improvement interventions; the engagement of teams in order to ensure that good practices are incorporated into care practice by overcoming the main obstacles and failure modes that directly interfere with reliable prophylaxis for risk patients; and the search for strategies and tools that can increase the chances of success through risk management and monitoring of multifaceted interventions.

The first and most important intervention of the project was to obtain the support of the strategic leadership of the health institutions and the leaders involved in this process. This action is automatically reflected in the prioritization of efforts, the availability of resources and the institutions' dedication to standardize processes. In the next step, we actively checked among the multidisciplinary team the status of interventions already implemented in order to understand what resources were available (structure, processes and people), what initiatives were in progress and the current performance of prophylaxis adequacy in the institution.

The education collaborative of this project offered support, support and education initiatives for the implementation of multidisciplinary interventions, making possible the alignment of processes as a fundamental basis for the validation stage of good practices in VTE prevention. The real-time monitoring of markers became one of the greatest challenges for institutions, given the imminent need to incorporate information technology aligned to clinical process data.

The primary objective of the project was to ensure that the practices and guidelines of international recommendations were carried out in a reliable manner and with multidisciplinary involvement. Our conceptual reference goes through the AHRQ reliability hierarchy that demonstrates the different stages of the multidisciplinary teams' efforts and the expected results for each phase of the process, as well as directing to a critical analysis regarding the institution's performance and the status of the implemented interventions. Each of the levels of the reliability hierarchy translates the performance regarding the level of adequate VTE prophylaxis (Table 11.5).

From this point on, the validation process promoted the timely management of the VTE prevention protocol in an effective way and supporting the development of resources and infrastructure to monitor and measure this work in the institutions based on five principles: process simplification, no interruption of the work flow, process reliability, small-scale intervention tests and monitoring of protocol use.

Table 11.5.   Levels of the VTE Prophylaxis Reliability and Performance Hierarchy.

Level	Description	Expected
1 'Natural' stage	No protocol	40%
2 'Pseudo' Protocol (the protocol exists, but is not managed)	No interface between prescriber and computerized system	50%
3 VTE Prevention Protocol	Protocol implemented and managed at the main points of care	65–85%
4 Strategies for leveraging the protocol	Reliability assessment of barriers	80–90%
5 VTE protocol integrated risk management	Identification of faults handled in real time	95% ou mais

Source: Maynard G. MD: Agency for Healthcare Research and Quality; August 2016. AHRQ Publication No. 16-0001-EF.

The institutions participating in this project had to meet the requirements of the eligibility criteria, among them:

1. To practice 'quality and safety' as the first priority within the organization.
2. To include VTE prevention among the strategic initiatives and policies for institutional security.
3. To have the support of senior management in the implementation of the improvement interventions in VTE prophylaxis.
4. To have the engagement of the clinical staff and multidisciplinary team in the implementation of the VTE protocol.
5. To have the VTE protocol described, updated and implemented, as well as this being one of the strategic focuses of the institution.
6. Manage the performance of VTE prophylaxis adequacy aligned to risk management.

Clinical, surgical and oncology patients were assessed, as well as verification standards, meeting the specificities of each profile. The subsequent stages are divided by practices addressing the following groupings:

Practice 1 – VTE Team: We objectively verified the degree of autonomy and involvement of the multidisciplinary team for the VTE prevention program, as well as its relationship with performance, satisfaction, safety, resource optimization and waste reduction. The role of the care leader was also analyzed, its dedication, establishment of goals and measurable objectives under the expected performance of VTE prophylaxis in the institution.

Practice 2 – VTE Prevention: Through this practice, it was possible to verify the robustness of the VTE protocol implemented in the care units in its entirety, its interface with the support processes (imaging diagnosis, clinical analysis and hemotherapy) and the main tracer points (periods of initial assessment and reassessment of VTE risk) according to the ARHQ process map. The standardization of a menu of therapeutic options, the management of bleeding risk through the register of contraindications to prophylaxis, were also fundamental items of analysis in this stage.

Practice 3 – Care Management: Priority in care management, we emphasized checking methods of assessment and application of drug and mechanical prophylaxis in a timely manner.

Practice 4 – Transition of Care: All care transition interfaces were considered regarding the effectiveness of multidisciplinary communication, communication with the patient, hospital discharge, adherence and compliance to VTE prophylaxis by higher-risk patients.

Practice 5 – Management of Complications: At this stage, we consider the standardization of a therapeutic management for cases of VTE, as well as the use of pharmacological antidotes when necessary.

Practice 6 – Risk Management: Immediate communication of complications and incidents was one of the crucial factors in the verification of expected performance. The use of digital technology in the search for failure modes and missed prevention opportunities and the monitoring of readmissions for VTE were among the most relevant interfaces for the management of care risk.

Practice 7 – Monitoring: In this stage, we verified the standardization and reliability of data collection to support the decision or review of interventions. In this sense, the use of systematized methods, such as clinical audit, were important support tools in monitoring the process.

The final phase of each monitoring cycle considered the sharing of prevention metrics, that is, process and result indicators as important management tools given their relevance in allowing the monitoring of the progress and impact of interventions.

Results

IBSP accompanied eight Brazilian institutions in this project, among medium and large hospitals, during two cycles of 12 months each. The operational model had a hybrid approach (face-to-face visits and videoconferencing) and was conducted by the technical scientific team of IBSP.

It was possible to support each of the institutions through educational actions targeted at the main failures to implement the multidisciplinary interventions found in the face-to-face visits and in conjunction with the use of the clinical audit tool (*tracer*). All the different opportunities for improvement identified in the institutions according to the structure of the project served as elements for structuring strategies for leveraging the protocol integrated to risk management and in the constant search for missed opportunities for prevention.

Conclusions

Patient safety research has taken directions to the incorporation of new disciplines never previously mapped as the behavioural psychology, the ergonomics, the communication, the theory of accidents and systems analysis. In the 21st century, patient safety began to become a specialized discipline in the field of education helping health professionals, managers, health organizations, politicians and citizens to adapt with the principles and concepts of the subject, because all of us may be affected one day.

The main aims of training in Patient Safety are to provide professionals with the skills to detect risks and factors that may contribute to patient safety incidents, but also to raise awareness of the whole team, including the patient, as the active participation of all in improving the safety of health care is essential.

The development and application of technology in the continuing education of health professionals is an important challenge and a good solution for continuing training. Health professions have been increasingly using simulation in the learning process of students and professionals, observing an evolution of technology as a resource for the continuing training of health professionals.

Digital technology and simulation should be used in health professions, supporting students and professionals to improve their clinical practices. The simulation of clinical cases promotes learning through error, in a virtual and controlled environment, facilitating reflection on practices, in safety. These training methodologies should be promoted as priority areas in Health Sciences Universities and Health Organisations, thus contributing to patient safety in health care.

Active Learning

Within the scope of education and training in patient safety some electronic resources may be used, namely, the IHI Open School courses provided by the Institute for Healthcare Improvement, of which we highlight:
'Quality Improvement Courses'

- QI 101: Introduction to Health Care Improvement
- QI 102: How to Improve with the Model for Improvement
- QI 103: Testing and Measuring Changes with PDSA Cycles
- QI 104: Interpreting Data: Run Charts, Control Charts, and Other Measurement Tools
- QI 105: Leading Quality Improvement
- QI 201: Planning for Spread: From Local Improvements to System-wide Change
- QI 202: Addressing Small Problems to Build Safer, More Reliable Systems

Available at https://www.ihi.org/education/ihi-open-school/Pages/courses-quality-improvement.aspx#QI101

Some websites provide videos that can be used in training contexts:Title: *Patient Safety Film:* https://www.youtube.com/watch?v=6YMZFRhh9L4

Title: *What is Quality Care?*: https://www.youtube.com/watch?v=erei6SZjcck
Title: *Speaking Up for Patient Safety*: https://www.youtube.com/watch?v=DCtGt
pkdC1U
The AHRQ has several courses and examples for training in patient safety: https://
psnet.ahrq.gov/continuing-education

References

Almeida, C. V. (2020). *Literacia em saúde e capacitação dos profissionais de saúde: O modelo de comunicação em saúde ACP*. Associação Portuguesa de Documentação e
Informação de Saúde. https://comum.rcaap.pt/handle/10400.26/34417

Costar, D. M., & Hall, K. K. (2020). Improving team performance and patient safety
on the job through team training and performance support tools: A systematic
review. *Journal of Patient Safety*, *16*(3S Suppl 1), S48–S56. https://doi.org/10.1097/
PTS.0000000000000746

Curtarelli, A., Silva, L. P. C. E., de Camargo, P. A. B., Pimenta, R. E. F., Jaldin, R. G.,
Bertanha, M., Sobreira, M. L., & Yoshida, W. B. (2019). Profilaxia de tromboembo-
lismo venoso, como podemos fazer melhor? Perfil de risco e profilaxia de trombo-
embolismo venoso em Hospital Universitário do interior do Estado de São Paulo.
Jornal Vascular Brasileiro, *18*. https://doi.org/10.1590/1677-5449.004018

Diniz, A. C., Bordalo, I., Ferreira, C., & Ramos, S. (2022). Mais letramento em saúde,
mais segurança do paciente: Um estudo de caso sobre campanhas de segurança do
paciente num centro hospitalar português. *Cadernos Ibero-Americanos de Direito
Sanitário*, *11*(3), 35–51. https://doi.org/10.17566/ciads.v11i3.917

Diniz, A. C., Ferreira, C. I., Damião, M. C., & Xavier, H. C. (2022). Health literacy of
oncologic patients and their informal caregivers: A pathway for patient safety. In C.
Vaz de Almeida & S. Ramos (Ed.), *Handbook of research on assertiveness, clarity,
and positivity in health literacy* (pp. 238–255). IGI Global. http://doi:10.4018/978-1-
7998-8824-6.ch014

Garcia, P., Cortez, B. C., & Sales, L. (2021). Simulação para a promoção da segurança do
doente. In F. Barroso, L. Sales, & S. Ramos (Coords.), *Guai Prático para a Segurança
do Doente* (pp. 343–350). Lidel-Edições Técnicas Lda.

Instituto Brasileiro para a Segurança do Paciente (IBSP). (2021). *Manual de validação de
boas práticas de segurança para prevenção do TEV* (2nd ed.). IBSP. ISBN: 978-65-
995674-0-7

Leotsakos, A., Ardolino, A., Cheung, R., Zheng, H., Barraclough, B., & Walton, M. (2014).
Educating future leaders in patient safety. *Journal of Multidisciplinary Healthcare*, *7*,
381–388. https://doi.org/10.2147/JMDH.S53792

Magalhães, T. (2021). Transformação Digital na Saúde. Contributos para a Mudança. In
T. Magalhães (Coord.), A. Santos (Direção Técnica). Editor: Almedina (1st ed.,
p. 494). ISBN: 978-989-40-0110-2

Maynard, G. (2016, August). *Preventing hospital-associated venous thromboembolism: A
guide for effective quality improvement* (2nd ed.). Agency for Healthcare Research
and Quality. AHRQ Publication No. 16-0001-EF.

Portugal. (2017). Despacho no. 6430/2017 Projeto-piloto «Literacia para a Segurança dos
Cuidados de Saúde. Diário da República: 2.a Série, No. 142 (25-07-2017), 15407-
15407. https://dre.pt/pesquisa/-/search/107744170/details/normal?l=1

Portugal. (2019). *Direção Geral da Saúde Segurança nos Cuidados de Saúde. Cursos Online*.
Plataforma NAU. http://www.usoresponsaveldomedicamento.com/landing/

Portugal. (2022). Ministério da Saúde. Direção-Geral da Saúde. Documento Técnico para a implementação do Plano Nacional para a Segurança dos Doentes 2021–2026. https://www.dgs.pt/documentos-e-publicacoes/plano-nacional-para-a-seguranca-dos-doentes-2021-2026-pdf.aspx

Ramos, S. (2020). Segurança do Doente e Literacia em Saúde. In C. V. Almeida, K. L. Moraes, & V. V. Brasil (Coords.), *50 Técnicas de literacia em saúde na prática. Um guia para a saúde* (Vol. 2, pp. 167–173).

Ramos, S., & Almeida, C. V. (2020). Speak up: Vitalizar o paciente para uma melhor literacia em saúde. In C. V. Almeida, K. L. Moraes, & V. V. Brasil (Coords.). *50 Técnicas de literacia em saúde na prática. Um guia para a saúde* (Vol. 2, pp. 190–194). http://www.chlc.min-saude.pt/wp-content/uploads/sites/3/2019/10/o-Central-3-Seguranca-Doente.pdf

Reis, C. T., Sousa, Isoppo, C. S., & Ramos, S. (2021). Formação Pós-graduada na area da segurança do paciente: Desafios e oportunidades. In *Qualidade no Cuidado e Segurança do Paciente: Educação, Pesquisa e Gestão* (Vol. 8, 1st ed., p. 500). Conselho Nacional de Secretários de Saúde – Conass.

Sousa, P., Uva, A. S., Serranheira, F., Uva, M. S., & Nunes, C. (2018). Patient and hospital characteristics that influence incidence of adverse events in acute public hospitals in Portugal: A retrospective cohort study. *International Journal for Quality in Health Care, 30*(2), 132–137. https://doi.org/10.1093/intqhc/mzx190

Stevenson, L., Lang, A., Macdonald, M., Archer, J. & Berlanda, C. (2012). Safety in home care: Thinking outside the hospital box. *Healthcare Quarterly, 15*(Spec No), 68–72. https://doi.org/10.12927/hcq.2012.22838. PMID: 22874450

Vincent, C., & Amalberti, R. (2015). Safety in healthcare is a moving target. *BMJ Quality & Safety, 24*(9), 539–540. https://doi.org/10.1136/bmjqs-2015-004403

Weaver, S. J., Dy, S. M., & Rosen, M. A. (2014). Team-training in healthcare: A narrative synthesis of the literature. *BMJ Quality & Safety, 23*(5), 359–372. https://doi.org/10.1136/bmjqs-2013-001848

World Health Organization (WHO). (2011). *Patient safety curriculum guide: Multiprofessional edition.* WHO. ISBN: 978-92-4-150195-8

World Health Organization (WHO). (2020). *Handbook for national quality policy and strategy: A practical approach for developing policy and strategy to improve quality of care.* WHO. ISBN: 978-92-4-000570-9

World Health Organization (WHO). (2021). *Global Patient Safety Action Plan 2021–2030: Towards eliminating avoidable harm in health care.* WHO. ISBN: 978-92-4-003270-5

Wu, A. W., & Busch, I. M. (2019). Patient safety: A new basic science for professional education. *GMS Journal for Medical Education, 36*(2), Doc21. https://doi.org/10.3205/zma001229

Chapter 12

The Economy and The Digital: Investments to Improve the Student Experience

*Eduardo Manuel de Almeida Leite[a,b,c] and
Ana Miguel Ramos Leite[c,d]*

[a] *University of Madeira, Madeira, Portugal*
[b] *CITUR-Madeira – Research Centre for Tourism Development and Innovation,
Madeira, Portugal*
[c] *OSEAN – Outermost Regions Sustainable Ecosystem for Entrepreneurship and
Innovation, Madeira, Portugal*
[d] *Faculty of Economics, University of Coimbra, Coimbra, Portugal*

Abstract

For several decades, universities have been trying to implement new technologies in their teaching methods, intending to create skills for the
twenty-first century. In the literature, this process is called digital transformation. This chapter is based on an integrative revision and solid work of the
authors in their university, providing students with technological devices,
such as laptops, tablets, and other gadgets to invest in digital education
skills. Concluding that investing in digital education is crucial for improving
the student experience and preparing students for the future workforce.

Keywords: Digital transformation; education; digital technologies;
active learning; communication; learning experience

1. Introduction

Educational institutions, in general, particularly universities, are central to the
creation of new knowledge-based economies. Digital technologies are key means
for realizing this potential (Selwyn, 2016).

Technology-Enhanced Healthcare Education:
Transformative Learning for Patient-Centric Health, 165–174
Copyright © 2024 by Eduardo Manuel de Almeida Leite and Ana Miguel Ramos Leite
Published under exclusive licence by Emerald Publishing Limited
doi:10.1108/978-1-83753-598-920231012

That's why, for several decades, universities have been trying to implement new technologies in their teaching methods, intending to create skills for the twenty-first century (JISC, 2017). In the literature, this process is called digital transformation. Digital transformation is understood as the formation of networks of actors in all segments of the value chain, with the integrated use of new technologies, also considering changes in talent, culture, and organizational structure (Farias-Gaytan et al., 2021).

In other words, the concept of digital transformation refers to a process that aims to introduce fundamental changes (revolution) in the internal and external functioning and relationships of organizations through the integration of various technologies. Like all other revolutionary changes, digital transformation involves intense adjustment/re-adjustment.

The profound changes in the socioeconomic education system resulting from the globalized economy (accelerated by the COVID-19 pandemic) have propelled changes specifically in higher education, such as education's standard, quality, decentralization, virtual, and independent learning (Mohamed Hashim et al., 2021).

As a rule, it is not easy to change paradigms. Certainly, for this reason, and despite the technological advances that have taken place in the field of education, there are still many challenges that need to be faced to integrate digital transformation into universities, namely, at the curriculum level.

An instance of this is how regional and global integration has enabled the advancement of education trends that encourage transnational education. As a result, digital education is emerging as a potential solution to bridge enrolment gaps, but this requires universities to adopt a proactive and entrepreneurial approach by providing learning programs in a shared language and preparing their human resources, such as lecturers and professors, for change.

However, this domain is arguably still in the infancy stage and differs in scope a lot, specifically examining the key benefits of digital transformation and its entrepreneurial capabilities from a university's perspective (Mohamed Hashim et al., 2021).

In this regard, the leadership of an educational institution should be accompanied by a technology-based strategy that emphasizes the development of skills and the use of digital tools (Beetham & Sharpe, 2023). To emphasize that, the focal point of digital transformation is not primarily the technological aspect but, rather, the strategic approach (Matt et al., 2015). According to UNESCO, this can be achieved by establishing a clear vision and a commitment to success. Obviously, this will facilitate the transformation of the teaching and learning experience, especially if lecturers' perception of how technology can be used in the classroom is positive in terms of ensuring scientific outcomes (Portuguez-Castro et al., 2022).

Indeed, in terms of university teaching perspectives, it is often said that they are the driving forces for implementing and developing digital teaching and learning, and, for this reason, technical as well as pedagogical guidance, is recommended (Pensel & Hofhues, 2017).

To sum up, the concept of digital transformation proposes a paradigm shift in how teaching is conducted to provide the best possible education to the students. It involves the use of technology in the learning environment. It requires the involvement of the lecturers and professors in the development of new proposals and simulations that will allow the testing of students' competencies. This involves the use of multiple tools and resources designed to help students develop their innovation skills. In addition to being able to provide the necessary tools and resources, educational institutions are also investing in the development of digital learning programs and curricula (Portuguez-Castro et al., 2022).

The primary objective of a university is knowledge development, and therefore, the digital transformation of higher education differs from digitalization in other domains. For instance, digital transformation in the business realm involves the creation of new business models, whereas, in the context of higher education, it pertains to the long-term economic and social impact of organizational change.

Hence, according to B. Bygstad et al. (2022), universities should adopt a learning-centric approach to digital transformation, that is, establish a shared learning space, integrating technologies, pedagogies, and organizational measures (Table 12.1). Professors and lecturers need to redefine their roles, moving from lecturing to orchestrating digital resources. Students should enhance their capacity to work in complex hybrid settings where different forms of digitalization take place.

Finally, the impact of technology in learning boils down to:

Table 12.1. Impacts of Technology in Learning.

Learning Experience	Impacts
Increased access to information	Advancements in technology have simplified the process of acquiring educational resources and information for students, regardless of whether they are in the classroom or beyond it. The internet, for instance, offers a plethora of educational resources, including textbooks, online courses, and educational videos, that students can access with ease
Personalized learning	The advent of technology has enabled customized learning experiences for students that cater to their distinct learning styles, interests, and requirements. As a result, it can lead to more engaging and effective learning experiences as students can progress at their own pace and concentrate on subjects that captivate their interest
Improved collaboration and communication	Technology has also made it easier for students to collaborate and communicate with each other, even when they are not in the same location. This can be especially valuable for students who are learning remotely, or for students who are working on group projects

(*Continued*)

Table 12.1. (*Continued*)

Learning Experience	Impacts
Increased engagement	Technology has the potential to increase student engagement by making learning more interactive, fun, and relevant. For example, students may be more likely to participate in class discussions or complete homework assignments if they are using technology that they find enjoyable and engaging
Access to real-world applications	Technology also provides students with access to real-world applications, simulations, and virtual experiences that can help to bring abstract concepts to life. This can make learning more engaging and meaningful, as students are able to see the real-world implications of what they are learning

2. Investments to Improve Student Experience

The integration of technology into education has been a major driving force behind changes in the way students learn and interact with course materials. The digital economy has opened new investment opportunities aimed at improving the student experience and preparing students for success in a rapidly changing world (World Economy Forum, 2016). In this essay, we will examine the different forms of investment in digital education and their potential impact on the student experience.

Providing students with technological devices such as laptops, tablets, and other gadgets is one of the principal forms of investment in digital education. This allows students to access course materials, conduct research, and complete assignments from anywhere. Such investments can have a substantial influence on student engagement and access to educational resources, as they can easily carry their learning materials with them. Additionally, the integration of technology in the classroom can lead to an interactive and engaging learning experience, as it enables students to participate in class discussions, work together with their peers, and access multimedia resources.

In addition to providing technological resources to students, investing in digital education also entails professional development for teachers (Margaryan, Littlejohn, & Vojt, 2011). This encompasses training on how to integrate technology effectively into their teaching, as well as guidance on the utilization of digital tools and platforms. Teachers who receive this type of professional development are better prepared to design engaging and effective learning experiences, as they can leverage technology to elevate their teaching and cater to the diverse needs of their students ((Beetham & Sharpe, 2023).

Investment in online course materials is another important aspect of digital education. This includes the development of digital textbooks, online resources, and interactive simulations, as well as the creation of massive open online courses (MOOCs) and other forms of online learning. Online course materials can help to improve access to educational resources, as students are able to access them from anywhere with an internet connection. Moreover, personalized learning experiences can be facilitated by online course materials, allowing students to concentrate on the topics that intrigue them and work at their own pace.

Investment in artificial intelligence (AI) is another area of growth in digital education. AI can be used to create more efficient and effective learning environments, including tutoring systems that use natural language processing and machine learning algorithms to provide personalized feedback and guidance to students. AI can also be used to analyze student data to identify areas of weakness and suggest targeted interventions, as well as to provide teachers with insights into student progress and engagement.

While investment in digital education has the potential to greatly improve the student experience, it is also important to consider issues of equity and access. The availability of technology is not uniform across all students, and investments in digital education must ensure that students from diverse backgrounds have equal prospects to leverage the benefits of technological advancements. This may include investments in infrastructure, such as broadband internet access and device distribution programs, as well as investments in professional development and training for teachers and students to ensure that they are equipped with the skills and knowledge they need to effectively use technology in the classroom.

While investment in digital education has the potential to greatly improve the student experience, there are also potential challenges and limitations to consider. For example, there may be concerns about the potential for increased screen time and decreased face-to-face interaction, as well as the potential for technology to distract students or interfere with the learning process (Wilson, Tete-Mensah, & Boateng, 2014). Furthermore, the expenses associated with technology, including the need for continuous support and maintenance, as well as ongoing professional development and training for teachers and students, could give rise to concerns.

3. Possibilities of Integrating Digital Skills in the Curriculum

It is the responsibility of teachers to encourage creativity, and facilitate opportunities for students to explore information, work collaboratively, think critically, solve problems, and create digital artefacts (Beetham & Sharpe, 2023). Universities integrate digital skills in their curriculum through cross-cutting and subject-based ICT teaching, internet skills, and office software in computer courses, assessed through exams and tests. Merely introducing digital literacy skills in schools is insufficient, and students should be exposed to them through scaffolding, embedded within the academic and professional context (Figure 12.1.). By including digital technologies in the curriculum, students can develop their thinking and expand their capabilities, fostering a more collaborative environment and reducing the time spent looking for remedial help outside of the learning environment

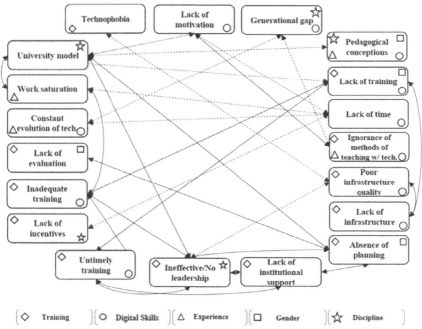

Fig. 12.1.   Explanatory Model of Barriers to Integration of Digital Technologies in University Teaching (MBIT). *Source*: Mercader (2020).

(Price-Dennis, Holmes, & Smith, 2015). Through online platforms, students can connect with their peers and experts, develop real-world connections, promote their projects, and receive feedback, enhancing their problem-solving and emotional intelligence skills (Armah & Van Der Westhuizen, 2020).

4. Concluding Remarks

The integration of technology in education has led to significant changes in the way students learn and interact with course material. The digital economy has created new opportunities for investment in education, aimed at improving the student experience and preparing them for the future workforce.

Investments in digital education have taken various forms, including the provision of laptops and other technology to students, development of online course materials, and training for teachers to effectively integrate technology into their teaching practice. The potential benefits of such investments include heightened student engagement, improved accessibility to educational resources, and personalized learning experiences.

Besides, there is a burgeoning interest in using advanced technologies, such as AI, to create a more efficient and effective learning environment. This includes the use of AI-powered tutoring systems, virtual and augmented reality, and data-driven insights to improve student performance and outcomes.

It is crucial to recognize that investments in digital education should address issues of fairness and access, given that not all students have equivalent access to technology. This implies that investments must be structured in a way that guarantees equal opportunities for students from all backgrounds to leverage the benefits of digital education advancements.

In conclusion, investment in digital education is crucial for improving the student experience and preparing students for the future workforce. However, it must be done in a way that addresses issues of equity and access and focuses on creating a high-quality learning environment that leverages technology to its full potential.

5. Active Learning Suggestions

5.1. Suggested Teaching Assignments

Creating and delivering a lesson plan that covers the following topics:

i.   *Introduction to digital education*: Explain what digital education is, its benefits, and its role in the modern education system.

ii.   *Types of digital education*: Discuss different types of digital education, such as online courses, distance learning, and blended learning.

iii. *Pros and cons of digital education*: Elaborate on the benefits of digital education, such as convenience and accessibility, while also examining the challenges, such as inequitable technology access and limited interaction with teachers and peers.

iv.   *Efficient utilization of technology in education*: Discuss the various types of technology that are used in digital education, such as learning management systems, virtual reality, and gamification, and how they can be used to enhance the learning experience.

v.   *Digital literacy and digital citizenship*: Emphasize the importance of digital literacy and explain what it entails, such as using technology effectively, evaluating information sources, and protecting online privacy.

vi.   *Optimal strategies in digital education*: Share best practices for teaching and learning in a digital environment, such as incorporating active learning strategies and providing clear guidelines and expectations for students.

vii. *Future of digital education*: Discuss the future of digital education and its potential impact on the education system, such as personalized learning and increased use of AI.

The assignment can include hands-on activities, group discussions, and a final project where students apply what they have learned to create a lesson plan of their own.

5.2. Recommended Readings

- Articles

  i   *United Nations – Assuring and improving quality public digital learning for all*: https://www.un.org/en/transforming-education-summit/digital-learning-all

  ii *Forbes – The future of education: How technology is transforming the classroom*: This article explores the ways in which technology is transforming education, including the use of online resources, virtual and augmented reality, and AI-powered tutoring systems.

  iii *EdTech Review – The digital divide in education: Challenges and opportunities –* This article discusses the digital divide in education and the challenges faced by students who do not have access to technology, as well as the opportunities that technology can provide for enhancing student learning and engagement.

- Video

  Bill Gates: how online courses can radically improve education by 2030 – https://youtu.be/Hrd0NiWMIjk

5.3. Case Study

Case Study: 'Digital Education in Rural School'
A small rural school in the midwestern United States has recently implemented a digital education program to supplement its traditional classroom curriculum. The program provides students with laptops and access to online resources, such as interactive lessons and virtual field trips. The school's goal is to prepare its students for the future workforce and to provide them with skills that are in demand, such as digital literacy and critical thinking.

Nevertheless, the school has encountered several difficulties in executing the initiative. Numerous students come from underprivileged families and do not have dependable internet access at home. Moreover, a few teachers have faced challenges in assimilating technology into their teaching style, given limited training on utilizing the digital tools provided.

Possible Discussion Questions:

- What steps can the school take to address the digital divide and ensure that all students have equal access to technology?
- How can the school provide ongoing training and support to teachers to help them effectively integrate technology into their teaching practice?
- What are the potential long-term benefits and drawbacks of implementing a digital education program in a rural school setting?

Titles for Research Essays

'Exploring the Student Experience in Online Learning: Perceptions and Outcomes'
'The Impact of Digital Education on Student Motivation and Engagement'

'The Use of Artificial Intelligence in Personalized Learning: Opportunities and Challenges'

'The Role of Digital Education in Promoting Economic Growth and Development'5.4

5.4. Recommended Projects URL

i   *OSEAN – Outermost Regions Sustainable Ecosystem for Entrepreneurship and Innovation*: https://osean.uma.pt

ii   *INCORE – Innovation Capacity Building for Higher Education in Europe's Outermost Regions*: https://incoreproject.eu

References

Armah, J. K., & Van Der Westhuizen, D. (2020). Embedding digital capability into the higher education curriculum: The case of Ghana. *Universal Journal of Educational Research, 8*(2), 346–354. https://doi.org/10.13189/ujer.2020.080203

Beetham, H., & Sharpe, R. (Eds.) (2013). An introduction to rethinking pedagogy. In *Rethinking pedagogy for a digital age* (pp. 25–36). Routledge.

Bygstad, B., Øvrelid, E., Ludvigsen, S., & dÆhlen, M. (2022). From dual digitalization to digital learning space: Exploring the digital transformation of higher education. *Computer Education, 182*, 104463. https://doi.org/10.1016/j.compedu.2022.104463

Farias-Gaytan, S., Aguaded, I., & Ramirez-Montoya, M. S. (2021). Transformation and digital literacy: Systematic literature mapping. *Education and Information Technologies, 27*, 1417–1437. https://doi.org/10.1007/s10639-021-10624-x

JISC. (2017). *Building digital capability*. https://www.JISC.ac.uk/rd/projects/building-digital-capability

Margaryan, A., Littlejohn, A., & Vojt, G. (2011). Are digital natives a myth or reality? University students' use of digital technologies. *Computers & Education, 56*(2), 429–440.

Matt, C., Hess, T., & Benlian, A. (2015). Digital transformation strategies. *Business & Information Systems Engineering, 57*(5), 339–343.

Mercader, C. (2020). Explanatory model of barriers to integration of digital technologies in higher education institutions. *Education and Information Technologies, 25*, 5133–5147.

Mohamed Hashim, M., Tlemsani, I., & Matthews, R. (2021). Higher education strategy in digital transformation. *Education and Information Technologies, 27*, 3171–3195. https://doi.org/10.1007/s10639-021-10739-1

Selwyn, N. (2016). Digital downsides: Exploring university students' negative engagements with digital technology. *Teaching in Higher Education, 21*(8), 1006–1021. https://doi.org/10.1080/13562517.2016.1213229

Pensel, S., & Hofhues, S. (2017). Digitale Lerninfrastrukturen an Hochschulen. Systematisches Review zu den Rahmenbedingungen für das Lehren und Lernen mit Medien an deutschen Hochschulen. Retrieved April 24, 2018, from http://your-study.info/wp-content/uploads/2018/01/Review_Pensel_Hofhues.pdf

Portuguez-Castro, M., Hernández-Méndez, R. V., & Peña-Ortega, L. O. (2022). Novus Projects: Innovative ideas to build new opportunities upon technology-based avenues in higher education. *Education Sciences, 12*, 695. https://doi.org/10.3390/educsci12100695

Price-Dennis, D., Holmes, K. A., & Smith, E. (2015). Exploring digital literacy practices in an inclusive classroom. *The Reading Teacher, 69*(2), 195–205.

Selwyn, N., & Facer, K. (2007). *Beyond the digital divide: Rethinking digital inclusion for the 21st century*. Futurelab.

Wilson, K. B., Tete-Mensah, I., & Boateng, K. A. (2014). Information and communication technology use in higher education: Perspectives from students. *European Scientific Journal, 10*(19), 239–241.

World Economy Forum. (2016). *The future of jobs employment, skills and workforce strategy for the Fourth Industrial Revolution*. http://www3. weforum.org/docs/WEF_Future_ of_Jobs.pdf

Chapter 13

The Flipped Classroom in Higher Education: A Bibliometric Review

Andreia de Bem Machado[a], Maria José Sousa[b] and Helena Belchior Rocha[b]

[a]Federal University of Santa Catarina, Florianópolis, Brazil
[b]ISCTE, Lisbon, Portugal

Abstract

Changes in the educational environment regarding the teaching–learning process are required as a result of social, economic, and cultural transitions. In light of this, this chapter will discuss and examine the flipped classroom method's qualities as well as potential applications for individualized higher education. A bibliometric review of the Scopus database would be done in order to fulfil the suggested goal, and a report on a flipped classroom's implementation at a Brazilian university was also provided. It was discovered that the traits are pre-class activities, actions done in preparation for class, and postclass activities. This instructional approach can be utilized to motivate pupils in individualized instruction.

Keywords: Flipped classroom; active methodology; higher education; problem-based learning; bibliometric review; pre-class activities

1. Introduction

The digital revolution has been fuelled by the social, political, cultural, academic, and technological transformations that have been taken place during the twenty-first century, including the globalization of business and information. As a result, the usage of digital information and communication technologies (DICT) in society increased significantly, bringing about large and quick changes in how people interact and communicate. There have been changes in the educational environment, particularly with regard to the teaching and learning process, in this technological context of changes in the way that information is received

Technology-Enhanced Healthcare Education:
Transformative Learning for Patient-Centric Health, 175–185
Copyright © 2024 by Andreia de Bem Machado, Maria José Sousa and Helena Belchior Rocha
Published under exclusive licence by Emerald Publishing Limited
doi:10.1108/978-1-83753-598-920231013

and communicated. These changes were made an effort to teach pupils critical thinking that was centred on the collective building of information in order to make it meaningful.

We may highlight the usage of technology as one of the primary developments in the educational environment (Mattar, 2018). Education has always made use of technology. The DICT, which is utilized for creating and disseminating knowledge, is among the several technologies that are currently present in the educational environment. This study emphasize, the flipped classroom approach as one of the varied ICT uses in education. By placing the student at the centre of the teaching–learning process, this methodology seeks to alter the logic of organizational structure in the classroom. This method gives the student access to the material that will be covered in class in advance, either through videos or other media. The student will use the time to further the subject matter through exercises and group projects when they are in sync with the teacher (Bergmann & Sams, 2012, 2015, 2016).

The results and discussions, or the bibliometric analysis, from the resultant scenario of scientific publications and the experience report are presented in the Section 4. The closing thoughts are presented in Section 6 before the references that were cited throughout the paper.

2. Flipped Classroom

Due to social changes, educational approaches have been changed to better match modern educational needs, with a stronger emphasis now being placed on the student as the main character in his own educational narrative. Flipped classroom is the term used to describe the approach described in this sentence. At the end of the 1990s, the phrase 'flipped classroom' was subsequently created (Baker, 2000). Early in 2007, American high school teachers Bergmann and Sams began to feel persistent dissatisfaction over their students' failure to apply what they learned in class to the homework that was given home. Bergman and Sams (2016) decided to record their lessons so that their pupils may view them at home as a result. They utilized the time in the classroom in this manner for debates and the confirmation of unclear topics. By active learning techniques including discussion, debate, and problem-solving, new knowledge was assimilated during class time. In this case, the classroom dynamics were altered by the use of technology to share questions and curiosities, placing the students in the teacher's former position as the centre of the teaching and learning process. The idea of the flipped classroom was created in this manner. Although this method of instruction has been studied since 2000, it was only with Professors Bergman and Sams that it became conceptualized in 2007. This method has some qualities that have been described by various authors and gained popularity during the pandemic that began in 2020 with the COVID-19 pandemic.

In a flipped classroom, students must finish their assignments before class in order to fully benefit from the synchronous work done in class during the active and social learning activities.

3. Methodology – Systematic Review

In order to increase knowledge, measure and analyze the publications scientific literature on trust in the flipped classroom theme and the possibilities of personalized teaching, a bibliometric analysis was performed, starting with a search in the Scopus (WoS) database by Clarivate Analytics. An approach with three phases – an execution plan, data collecting, and bibliometrics – was used to create the study. The bibliometrix program was utilized to examine the bibliometric data because it is most compatible with the Scopus database. Among the tools for bibliometric analysis that have been studied, the R Bibliometrix package Biblioshiny provides a comprehensive and suitable collection of approaches (Moral-Muñoz et al., 2020). This data allowed for the grouping of pertinent information for bibliometric analysis, including temporal distribution, major authors, institutions, and countries, kind of publishing in the field, keywords, and articles with the highest citations. Scientific mapping enables one to look into and create a statistically based global image of scientific knowledge. It primarily presents the structural and dynamic features of a scientific investigation using the three knowledge frameworks.

The study is categorized as exploratory-descriptive in order to characterize the theme and develop the familiarity of researchers with the issue in order to solve the problem of this research. The study is classified as exploratory-descriptive with the aim of characterizing the topic and developing researcher familiarity with the issue in order to answer the problem of this research. The study was divided into two phases: bibliometrics and the experience report.

An online database was thoroughly searched, and the findings of the search were then subjected to a bibliometric study. A method used in information science called bibliometrics maps materials based on bibliographic records that are kept in databases using mathematical and statistical techniques (Linnenluecke et al., 2019). Among other pertinent findings, bibliometrics enables the systematization of research findings and the reduction of biases that can occur when analyzing a given topic. These findings include the number of productions by region, the temporality of publications, the organization of research by field of knowledge, the count of literature related to the study's citations, and the impact factor of a scientific publication. The study was divided into three independent phases for the bibliometric analysis: planning, data collecting, and findings. These steps came together in order to respond to the study's central question, which was: What are the characteristics of the flipped classroom? The research was completed in December 2022, after planning had finished in September. Due to the quantity of documents deemed sufficient in the Web search bases, some criteria were specified in this phase, such as restricting the search to electronic databases and excluding physical library catalogues. Due to the Scopus database's importance in the academic setting and its interdisciplinary nature, which is the emphasis of study in this field, it was specified as important to the research domain in the planning scope. This was done in addition to the fact that it is one of the biggest databases of bibliographic references and abstracts of works of science that have undergone peer review.

4. Analysis of the Selected Publications

The search terms 'Inverted Class' OR 'Inverted Classroom' AND 'Flipped Classroom' 'concept' were defined when the research was still in the planning stages. The Boolean operator OR was used to incorporate as many papers as possible that deal with the research's main issue. To improve the outcome of the literature search for 'flipped classroom' and its writing variations, the truncator (*) was used. As a concept depends on the context to which it is related, it is believed that the variations of the expressions employed in the search are provided, in a bigger context, inside the same proposal. Lastly, it was chosen to just use the terms defined in the 'title, abstract, and keyword' sections when planning the search, excluding any additional criteria that would have limited the results, such as time or language. In the planning phase, to meet the research problem: What are the characteristics of the flipped classroom? The following search terms were used: 'Inverted Class' OR 'Inverted Classroom' AND 'Flipped Classroom' 'concept', which was originated from 30 documents. From the research planning, data collection retrieved a total of 307 indexed papers, which indicated records from 2012

Table 13.1.   Summary of the Information Found in the Databases.

Description	Results
Main Information About Data	
Timespan	2012:2022
Sources (Journals, Books, etc.)	24
Documents	30
Annual growth rate %	-6,7
Document average age	5,77
Average citations per doc	41,53
References	1
Document Contents	
Keywords Plus (ID)	174
Authors	
Authors	89
Authors of single-authored docs	7
Authors Collaboration	
Single-authored docs	7
Co-authors per doc	3.1
International co-authorships %	23.33

Table 13.1.   (*Continued*)

Description	Results
Document Types	
Article	12
Book chapter	1
Conference paper	15
Editorial	1
Review	1

Source: Prepared by the authors (2023).

(the first publication) to 2022. As a result of this collection, it was identified that these papers were written by 89 authors, linked to 50 institutions from 14 different countries, and 174 keywords were used. Table 13.1 shows the results of this data collection in a general bibliometric analysis.

Eligible articles in the Scopus database were published between 2012 and 2022. Among these 30 articles, there is a varied list of authors, institutions, and countries that stand out in research on the flipped classroom and the possibilities of personalized teaching. When analyzing the 14 countries with the most publications in the area, it is clear that Germany stands out, with an average of 24% of the total number of publications, totaling 15 articles. In second place USA, with 22% of publications, as shown in Fig. 13.1:

Another analysis performed is related to the identification of authors. Among the authors who have more production on the flipped classroom and personalized

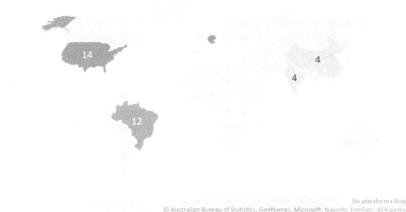

Da plataforma Bing
© Australian Bureau of Statistics, GeoNames, Microsoft, Navinfo, TomTom, Wikipedia

Fig. 13.1.   Country Distribution of the Papers. *Source*: Prepared by the authors (2023).

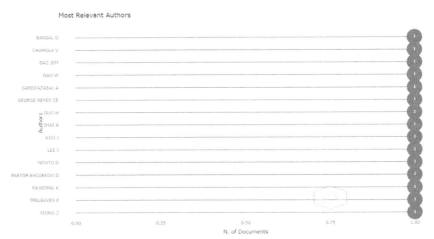

Fig. 13.2.   Most Relevant Authors. *Source*: Prepared by the authors (2023).

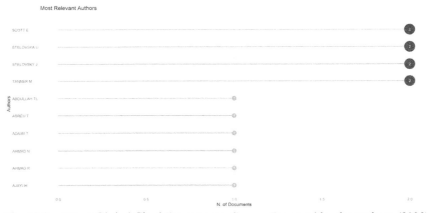

Fig. 13.3.   Most Global Cited Documents. *Source*: Prepared by the authors (2023).

learning, we highlight E. Scott, U. Stelovska, J. E. Stelovsky, and M. Tanner, with two publications, as shown in Fig. 13.2:

The paper that gained prominence with 842 citations was how learning in an Inverted Classroom influences cooperation, innovation, and task orientation by authors S. Jeremy and F. Strayer published in the year 2012, as shown in Fig. 13.3.

The hierarchy of the research sub-branches in the fields of flipped classrooms and personalized learning could also be analyzed from the overall survey. The collection of rectangles used to illustrate the TreeMap, as seen in Fig. 13.4, proportionally displays the hierarchy of the research's sub-branches. It is clear that topics like teaching and student education make an appearance with some relevance and have something to do with the flipped classroom.

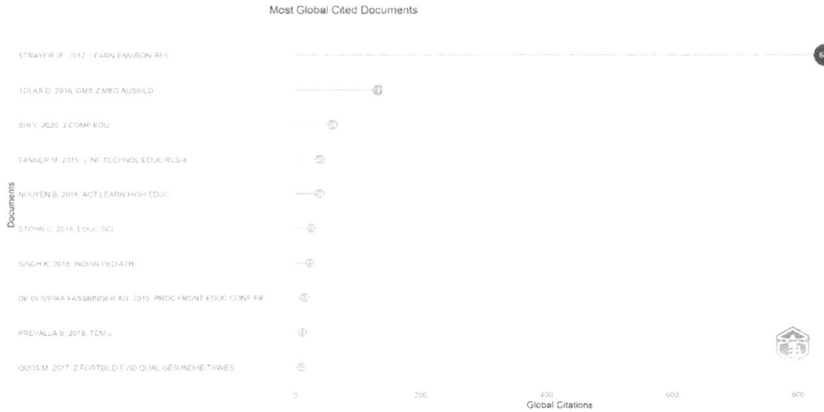

Most Global Cited Documents

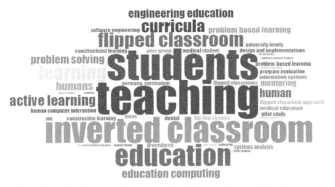

Fig. 13.4.   TreeMap. *Source*: Prepared by the authors (2023).

Fig. 13.5.   Tag Cloud. *Source*: Prepared by the authors (2023).

The 'cloud of words' was created using bibliometric analysis, based on the data the work group recovered, using 174 key terms that the authors had picked. The word 'teaching' appeared in the sequence's highlight 16 times in total. 'Students' came in second. Fig. 13.5 extended the tag cloud, which displays the essential terms, was created using this data.

In the bibliometric review, it was found that the countries discuss this theme the most are: Germany stands out in first place, with an average of 24% of the total number of publications, totaling 15 articles; and USA in second place, with 22% of publications. Nãoháautorreferênciasobre o tema. The paper that gained prominence with 842 citations was 'How Learning in an Inverted Classroom Influences Cooperation, Innovation and Task Orientation' (2012) by S. Jeremy and F. Strayer.

5. Experience Report

Inverted Classroom, also known as flipped classroom, is an educational model where students are first introduced to the course material through pre-recorded lectures, readings, or other resources, and then they attend the class to work on activities, projects, and discussions related to the topic. The model has gained attention in recent years as a student-centred approach that allows for more inter-action, engagement, and personalized learning. In 2022, I had the opportunity to implement the Inverted Classroom model in a graduation course at a university in Brazil, and I would like to share my experience in light of the research conducted by Hendrik and Hamzah (2021) and González and Gaytán (2019).

Three classes used the inverted class dynamic in the synchronous and asynchronous digital teaching mode (supported by the Moodle virtual environment) in 2020 and 2021: 2020–2021, 2020–2022, and 2021–2021. There were roughly 50 pupils present in each lesson.

In Moodle, all of the instructional material was organized into modules:

1. *Attendance* – the location where students can sign up for the synchronous class.
2. Access to the classroom via a link.
3. *Activities and Script Delivery*: A script defining the topics to be covered in each synchronous class, the students' tasks for the asynchronous class, and the due dates for the evaluation activities was made accessible in this case.
4. Each chapter of the textbook used in the discipline has its own module, which includes a video with the chapter's content, a pdf of the chapter, and supplementary readings and videos.

The instructional strategies employed in the sessions included both solo and team exercises (composed of 5–6 students), with the first aiming to encourage self-learning and self-reflection on the part of the student and the latter to foster teamwork and discussion. Each student had to read the text or view the video lesson in order to complete the mind map assignment, which required them to create one for each chapter of the book.

The debate in class took place in the theoretical-applied synchronous classes, where the teacher sparked it by asking the students to apply their knowledge to real-world situations. Students should present instances of systems and characterize them using the systemic perspective when studying the notion of systems, for instance.

It was also adopted the problem-based methodology, which we called an Integrative Project, in which each team should select a real problem of low complexity (but not trivial), and describe it with a systemic and critical look in accordance with what was learned in class and the tools that were presented, such as problem maps, root causes, empathy maps, interviews with those who experienced the problem, with the idea being that they truly understood the problem and developed a systemic approach. Each team's preliminary findings from this process were presented in class or in the forum, where they received comments from their peers and teachers.

Before the course started, I recorded video lectures and created online quizzes and discussion forums for each topic. I also provided readings and other resources, such as podcasts and videos, to complement the lectures. Students were required to watch the videos, complete the quizzes, and participate in the forums before coming to class. During the face-to-face meetings, we used active learning strategies, such as group discussions, case studies, and simulations, to deepen the understanding of the topics and apply the concepts to real-world situations.

The implementation of the Inverted Classroom model resulted in several benefits. Firstly, students were more engaged in the learning process, as they had the opportunity to prepare for the classes and come up with questions and doubts. This increased their participation and interaction during the face-to-face meetings and facilitated the development of critical thinking and problem-solving skills. As Hendrik and Hamzah (2021) noted, 'the flipped classroom approach is an effective strategy for promoting student engagement and active learning'.

Secondly, the Inverted Classroom model allowed for a more personalized approach to learning, as students could watch the videos and work on the quizzes at their own pace, and then focus on the topics that were more challenging during the classes. This approach promoted self-directed learning and autonomy, and helped students to take ownership of their learning process. González Fernández argues that 'flipped learning enables teachers to personalize learning for their students and create opportunities for student-centred, inquiry-based instruction'.

Lastly, the Inverted Classroom model allowed for more time for active learning during the face-to-face meetings, as the lectures were delivered online. This approach provided more opportunities for collaborative learning and peer-to-peer interactions, which helped to develop communication and teamwork skills.

In conclusion, the Inverted Classroom model proved to be a successful approach to teaching a graduation course at a university in Brazil. The model promoted engagement, personalized learning, and active learning, and allowed for more time for collaborative and peer-to-peer interactions during the face-to-face meetings. The research conducted by Hendrik and Hamzah (2021) and González and Gaytán (2019), supports the effectiveness of the Inverted Classroom model in promoting student-centred and inquiry-based learning, and suggests that this approach can lead to increased academic achievement and social skills development.

6. Final Considerations

The result is that the USA and Germany are the two nations that publish the most on this topic. E. Scott, U. Stelovska, J. E. Stelovsky, and M. Tanner are the authors who have produced the most material on the flipped classroom and personalized learning. 'How Learning in an Inverted Classroom Influences Cooperation, Innovation, and Task Orientation' (2012) was the study that attracted the most attention, receiving 842 citations, written by S. Jeremy and F. Strayer.

The flipped classroom's major characteristics are that it is a teaching method where videos take the role of direct instruction, and in actual classrooms, students are encouraged to concentrate on crucial learning tasks alongside their teachers. By acquiring strategies for taking a lot of knowledge, it is an educational innovation that enables pupils to improve their critical thinking abilities. This lesson plan includes a video tutorial that may be seen outside of the classroom. It is a tactic for enhancing communication and learning abilities as well as for producing and distributing knowledge that may be incorporated.

The flipped classroom primarily consists of in-class activities, which refer to the interactive environment that relies on learning based on teamwork, lab activities, peer instruction, collaborative learning, and problem-based critical thinking, as well as out-of-class activities, which refer to the time used by students preparing for classroom activities, reading a textbook, and watching a slide presentation.

The idea behind the 'flipped classroom', as it is described in the experience report, is to encourage collaboration between students and teachers in order to make learning more engaging and personalized in the classroom environment.

It is found that the flipped classroom strategy used in this research worked well for individualized learning and helped students acquire a wide range of knowledge. The students understood the value of communication, teamwork, and time management in addition to the theoretical material of the course and were able to apply it to their professional lives.

The subject still requires a lot of research; therefore, for upcoming projects, we advise looking into how the flipped classroom might assess students' development.

References

Baker, J. W. (2000). *The classroom flip: Using web course management tools to become the guide by the side*. Selected papers from the 11th international conference on college teaching and learning.

Bergmann, J., & Sams, A. (2012). *Flip your classroom: Reach every student in every class every day*. International Society for Technology in Education.

Bergmann, J., & Sams, A. (2015). *Flipped learning for science instruction*. International Society for Technology in Education.

Bergmann, J., & Sams, A. (2016). *Sala de Aula Invertida*. Uma Metodologia Ativa de Aprendizagem. LTC.

González Fernández, M. O., & Gaytán, P. H. (2019). Experiencia del aula invertida para promover estudiantesprosumidoresdelnivel superior. *Revista Iberoamericana de Educación a Distancia, 22*(2), 245.

Hendrik, H., & Hamzah, A. (2021). Flipped classroom in programming course: A systematic literature review. *International Journal of Emerging Technologies in Learning, 16*(02), 220.

Linnenluecke, M. K., Marrone, M., & Singh, A. K. (2019). Conducting systematic literature reviews and bibliometric analyses. *Australian Journal of Management*, 031289621987767.

Mattar, J. (2018). Constructivism and connectivism in education technology: Active, situated, authentic, experiential, and anchored learning/El constructivismo y el conectivismoentecnologíaeducativa: El aprendizajeactivo, situado, auténtico, experiencial y anclado. *Revista Iberoamericana de Educación a Distancia*, *21*(2), 201–217. https://doi.org/10.5944/ried.21.2.2005

Moral-Muñoz, J. A., Herrera-Viedma, E., Santisteban-Espejo, A., & Cobo, M. J. (2020). Software tools for conducting bibliometric analysis in science: An up-to-date review. *El Profesional de la Información*, *29*(1), e290103.

Saint-Onge, M. (1999). *O ensino na escola*. Edições Loyola.

Chapter 14

Transformative Learning as a bold Strategy for the Vision 2030 in Saudi Arabia: Moving Higher Healthcare Education Forward

Basim S. Alsaywid[a], Sarah Abdulrahman Alajlan[a] and Miltiadis D. Lytras[b]

[a]Saudi National Institute of Health, Riyadh, Saudi Arabia
[b]Effat University, Jeddah, Saudi Arabia

Abstract

The impact of education and research skills on the strategic digital transformation of education is straightforward. In this context, the Saudi National Institute of Health plays a pivotal role in the design and implementation of a resilient and robust strategy for the development of skills and competencies to young health professionals. In this chapter, the authors provide a brief overview of the Vision 2030 in Saudi Arabia and its basic priorities in the areas related to the Education and Research in the healthcare domain. The authors also elaborate on the key plans and initiatives undertaken by the education and research skills directory of the Saudi National Institute of Health (SNIH) towards transformative learning with impact on the implementation of the Vision 2030.

Keywords: Transformative learning; Digital Transformation in Healthcare; Saudi National Institute of Health; Vision 2030, Saudi Arabia; research and development; skills and competencies management

Technology-Enhanced Healthcare Education:
Transformative Learning for Patient-Centric Health, 187–207
Copyright © 2024 by Basim S. Alsaywid, Sarah Abdulrahman Alajlan and Miltiadis D. Lytras
Published under exclusive licence by Emerald Publishing Limited
doi:10.1108/978-1-83753-598-920231014

1. Introduction

Saudi Arabia is currently undergoing a comprehensive transformation program aimed at achieving a prosperous and dynamic society, a thriving economy, and an ambitious nation. The Vision 2030 plan, initiated by the government, aims to unlock the full potential of the Kingdom's people and resources, with a focus on its citizens and the Islamic religion. The vision includes a range of strategic objectives, such as expanding cultural and entertainment opportunities within the kingdom, encouraging healthy lifestyles, and developing the nation's infrastructure (Chowdhury et al., 2021; Saudi Vision 2030, 2023).

One of the key objectives of the Vision 2030 plan is to diversify the economy and create exciting job possibilities for the people of Saudi Arabia. This will be achieved through a focus on education, entrepreneurship, and innovation. The country will diversify its economy by privatizing state-owned assets, including the establishment of a sovereign wealth fund, which will be financed through partial initial public offering. The government will also open up underdeveloped sectors like manufacturing, renewable energy, and tourism (Saudi Vision 2030, 2023).

In order to achieve these objectives, the curriculum and standards of Saudi educational institutions will be modernized, starting from early childhood. This includes a focus on developing a highly skilled and innovative workforce that can drive the country's economic growth. To this end, the government has set a target of having at least five Saudi universities among the world's top 200 universities by 2030 (Mohiuddin et al., 2023).

Higher education in Saudi Arabia has undergone significant changes over the past decade. In 2013, the Ministry of Education launched an initiative aimed at improving the quality of higher education in the Kingdom. The initiative, known as the National Commission for Academic Accreditation and Assessment (NCAAA), has worked to enhance the quality of higher education by establishing national academic standards and accrediting universities and academic programs (Al Bu Ali et al., 2013; Mohiuddin et al., 2023).

In addition, the government has increased its investment in higher education, including funding for research and development initiatives. The goal is to position Saudi Arabia as a global leader in research and innovation with a focus on areas, such as energy, healthcare, and biotechnology (Alfawaz et al., 2022).

Overall, the Vision 2030 plan represents a significant opportunity for the people of Saudi Arabia. By investing in education, entrepreneurship, and innovation, the Kingdom can create a thriving economy and a vibrant society. With a focus on modernizing the curriculum and standards of Saudi educational institutions, the country can create a highly skilled and innovative workforce that can drive the country's economic growth.

2. Overview of Transformative Learning

Saudi Arabia's Vision 2030 is a bold and ambitious plan to build a stronger, more prosperous future for the Kingdom. A key area of focus under this initiative is transformative learning, which is seen as fundamental to creating new job opportunities and fostering career growth for Saudi students. To this end, a large number of scholarships have been granted to Saudi students to pursue studies in different fields, supplementing domestic bursaries to broaden access to high-quality education (Al-Hanawi et al.. 2019; Alsanosi, 2022).

Through transformative learning, Saudi Arabia aims to prepare its young people for the challenges and opportunities of the twenty-first century. This involves creating a more dynamic and inclusive education sector that encourages critical thinking, creativity, and problem-solving skills. Initiatives like the Saudi Digital Academy and Digital Innovation Labs are examples of how the government is investing in the development of the country's technological capabilities, nurturing the talents and skills of Saudi youth in collaboration with the private sector (Al-Rabiah Highlights Updates of Transformation Programs and Initiatives 2020 Saudi Ministry of Health, 2019; Smart Government Strategy in the Kingdom of Saudi Arabia; Uddin & Alharbi, 2023).

By promoting transformative learning, Saudi Arabia hopes to provide young people with the tools they need to succeed in whatever career they choose. This includes cultivating values such as social responsibility and ethical decision making, which are crucial for building a prosperous and equitable society. Through education, entrepreneurship, and innovation, the Kingdom seeks to create new opportunities for its people, while promoting economic growth and sustainability.

Moving higher education forward is a key component of the Vision 2030 plan in Saudi Arabia. By emphasizing the importance of transformative learning, the government is signalling its commitment to creating a more dynamic and forward-looking education sector. Through public–private partnerships and strategic investments, Saudi Arabia is working to establish itself as a leader in research and development, while also creating new pathways to career success and personal fulfilment. Ultimately, the success of the Vision 2030 plan will depend on the ability of the Kingdom to create a culture of lifelong learning, in which young people are empowered to tap into their potential and become drivers of their own futures.

2.1. Definitions and Theories of Transformative Learning

Transformative learning is a process of deep and meaningful personal and social change that can occur through education, critical reflection, and dialogue (Vipler et al., 2021). It involves a shift in perspective or worldview that can lead to new ways of thinking and acting, and a sense of empowerment and agency. This approach to learning is particularly relevant to the Vision 2030 plan in Saudi Arabia, which aims to create a more dynamic, innovative, and resilient society through education, entrepreneurship, and innovation.

The COVID-19 pandemic has been a major catalyst for transformative learning in Saudi Arabia, particularly in the higher education sector (Khalil et al., 2020). When universities were forced to close due to the pandemic, they quickly pivoted to online learning, leveraging innovative technologies to deliver virtual classes and maintain continuity of learning (Vipler et al., 2022). This was made possible in part by the world-class module platform, which allowed students from different universities in the Kingdom to access specific modules tailored to their needs.

This transition to online learning was a defining moment for the higher education sector in Saudi Arabia, and it opened up new opportunities for transformative learning. By breaking down traditional barriers to learning, such as physical location and time constraints, online learning has made it possible for more people to access high-quality education and training. This is particularly important for Saudi Arabia, which is seeking to create a more dynamic and innovative workforce that is ready to compete in the global marketplace (Hassounah et al., 2020).

At the heart of transformative learning is the idea that learning is a collaborative and dialogic process that involves questioning assumptions, challenging beliefs, and exploring diverse perspectives (Reay & Collier, 2017). This involves creating a safe and supportive learning environment in which individuals feel free to express themselves and engage with others in a spirit of mutual respect and understanding. By promoting such a learning environment, Saudi Arabia can create a culture of lifelong learning and personal growth that can drive economic development and social progress.

Several theories and models have been developed to describe the transformative learning process. One such framework is Mezirow's transformative learning theory, which proposes that personal and social change can occur through a process of critical reflection on one's assumptions and beliefs, and the creation of new meaning and perspective through dialogue and action (Eschenbacher & Fleming, 2020). Another model, developed by Cranton, emphasizes the role of emotions and identity in transformative learning, arguing that learners need to engage with their feelings, values, and sense of self in order to make meaningful and lasting change (Cranton, 1994; Taylor & Tisdell, 2017).

2.2. Benefits of Transformative Learning in Higher Education

Transformative learning has the potential to bring a range of benefits to higher education in Saudi Arabia, from increased learner engagement to enhanced critical thinking and innovation. By promoting a more dynamic and interactive learning environment, transformative learning can help to prepare students for the challenges and opportunities of the twenty-first century, while also fostering personal growth and social progress.

One of the key benefits of transformative learning is that it can lead to deeper engagement and motivation among learners. By encouraging students to take an active role in their learning, rather than simply absorbing information passively, transformative learning can create a sense of personal ownership and investment in the learning process. This can lead to more sustained effort and higher levels of achievement, as well as broader transferable skills like resilience and self-motivation (Magkoufopoulou, 2023).

Transformative learning can also lead to the development of critical-thinking skills, which are critical to success in higher education and beyond (Akköse et al., 2023). By encouraging learners to question assumptions, challenge beliefs, and explore diverse perspectives, transformative learning can create a more open-minded and intellectually curious community of learners. This can lead to more creative and innovative problem solving, as well as more effective communication and collaboration across different disciplines and sectors.

Another potential benefit of transformative learning is that it can help to cultivate a culture of innovation and entrepreneurship in higher education (Fisher-Yoshida et al., 2009). By encouraging students to think outside the box, take risks, and experiment with new approaches, transformative learning can create a more dynamic and responsive learning environment that is better able to adapt to the changing needs of the economy and society. This can lead to new opportunities for career growth and professional development, as well as social and economic progress on a broader level.

3. The Vision 2030 and Higher Education in Saudi Arabia

The Vision 2030 plan calls for the transformation of Saudi Arabia's economy and society, with a priority on improving the country's education system. Higher education in Saudi Arabia is expected to undergo significant changes in the coming years as a result of the Vision 2030 plan, with both challenges and opportunities for transformational change (Bataeineh & Aga, 2022).

One of the main opportunities presented by the Vision 2030 plan is the integration of digital technology into higher education (Alfahad, 2012; Alotaibi, 2022). With the COVID-19 pandemic and changing times, technology has become an essential aspect of education globally. This shift provides higher education institutions in Saudi Arabia with the chance to enhance their program offerings and improve the quality of education provided to students. Making the shift to digital education can also bring about cost efficiencies, flexible learning options for students, and an improved overall learning experience. Moreover, it can open up Saudi Arabia's higher education sector to global opportunities of both teaching and enrolment, as international students can now study in their native country without physically being present (Alasmari, 2023; Alebaikan & Troudi, 2010).

However, the integration of digital technology into higher education is not without its challenges (Duhaney, 2005). Financially, integrating educational activities and programs with technology can be costly and may not generate expected revenue or donations, especially concerning building new platforms to cater to a massive number of participants at the same time. This requires institutions to carefully plan and budget for the costs of transition to digital. The legal implications of intellectual property and accreditation issues also pose a significant risk that needs to be addressed. Operational challenges such as technical failure or supply chain disruptions are also a potential headache to deal with. Resistance from faculty and students can also put a strain on the transition process, particularly for those who are more comfortable with traditional teaching methods (Strecker et al., 2018).

Nonetheless, there is potential for solutions to overcome these challenges. It is important to prepare and be ready for any obstacles that may arise. Financial planning and strategic partnerships with tech service providers can ensure a smoother journey. Developing sound legal frameworks with intellectual property experts and adhering to guidelines laid out to protect intellectual property can prevent legal battles. Operational challenges can be mitigated through proper investment in technological infrastructure and backup procedures. Faculty and student resistance can be mitigated through training and awareness programs.

The Vision 2030 plan offers opportunities for higher education in Saudi Arabia to transform and adapt to changing times. Digitizing higher education and integrating technology comes with challenges, but adequate planning and preparedness are essential elements that can help mitigate these challenges. Addressing challenges and capitalizing on opportunities can improve the quality and accessibility of higher education in Saudi Arabia, as well as put the country in a favourable position to compete in the global education market.

3.1. Overview of The Vision 2030 Plan and Its Goals for Education

The Vision 2030 plan is an ambitious long-term plan put forth by the Kingdom of Saudi Arabia aimed at diversifying its economy, developing its society, and reducing its dependence on oil (Nurunnabi, 2017). A significant part of this plan is centred around improving the education system in Saudi Arabia, with a focus on enhancing the quality of education and aligning it with the needs of the modern-day labour market (Thompson, 2017).

One of the key objectives of the Vision 2030 plan for education is to create equality between graduates and the needs of the labour market (Alharbi & Alshammari, 2020). The goal is to bridge the gap between education and employment and to ensure that graduates are equipped with the skills and knowledge necessary to succeed in the job market. Additionally, the plan aims to develop the capabilities and skills of students in various educational stages to better prepare them for the workforce (Alesawi et al., 2023; Mitchell & Alfuraih, 2018).

Another goal is to increase the quality of qualified graduates for employment and scientific research. Saudi Arabia seeks to improve the quality of education and research in order to encourage innovation and entrepreneurship. Five Saudi universities are targeted to be listed among the world's top 200 universities by 2030, demonstrating the country's commitment to providing higher-quality education (Al-Youbi et al., 2021; Shahwan & Zaman, 2023).

In an effort to create a supportive environment for innovation, the Vision 2030 plan also works to encourage creators and innovators. Programs aimed at guiding students towards careers and professions that match their abilities and interests will help foster a culture of innovation and creativity.

The area of scientific research is receiving significant attention under the Vision 2030 plan. The SNIH was established in 2020 to provide opportunities for those interested in research to learn and practice more about research. The Research, Development and Innovation Authority (RDIA) coordinates activities of institutions and scientific research centrs, proposes policies, legislation and regulations, and provides financing related to the sector that matches with 2030 vision. This initiative not only promotes research activities but also provides opportunities for scholarships in research.

3.2. Current State of Higher Education in Saudi Arabia

The higher education system in Saudi Arabia has made significant progress since its inception, with an increasing number of students enrolled in universities and colleges across the country (Alamri, 2011). However, while there are certain strengths to the current system, it also has some weaknesses that need to be addressed to achieve the long-term goals set forth in the Vision 2030 plan (Al-Hanawi et al., 2020; Alharbi, 2016; Bin Othayman, et al., 2022; Smith & Abouammoh, 2013).

One of the strengths of the higher education system in Saudi Arabia is its emphasis on Islamic education, which is deeply ingrained in the country's culture and tradition. Another strength is the availability of scholarships and financial aid, which have helped many students pursue higher education in the country and abroad. The country's extensive investment in higher education infrastructure and modernization efforts has also helped to improve the quality of education offered in universities and colleges.

Despite these strengths, the higher education system in Saudi Arabia faces several challenges and weaknesses. One of the most significant challenges is the lack of collaboration between universities and the private sector. There is a need for greater coordination and communication between universities and businesses to ensure that the skills and knowledge being taught in higher education institutions align with the needs of the modern-day labour market.

The quality of education imparted also needs improvement, to create a more holistic and practical approach to learning. There is also a need for more research and development activities in higher education institutions. Currently, research and development activities are limited, and there is little emphasis on attracting top faculty and researchers to the country.

Another challenge is the limited opportunities for women in higher education. While there has been progress made in this area, female enrolment in higher education remains low compared to males. Inflexible traditional gender roles still present obstacles for women to enrol or put-in fully in educational activities, such as teacher training, STEM fields, or professional tracks.

A lack of transparency and accountability in academic programs and educational outcomes is another challenge. It can be difficult to evaluate the effectiveness of higher education institutions and their programs due to a lack of benchmarking, peer review mechanisms, or policy evaluation that creates confusion in academic recognition.

There is a need for significant improvements to the higher education system in Saudi Arabia to achieve the goals set forth in the Vision 2030 plan. To address the challenges and weaknesses discussed, there must be a more comprehensive collaboration between academic institutions and the private sector, investment in research and development, and a more practical approach to learning. Additionally, there should be more emphasis on attracting and retaining top faculty and researchers, and increased opportunities for women in higher education, by making necessary means to support the same. Likewise, creating evaluation mechanisms for academic programs outcomes is important for transparency and accountability.

3.3. Challenges and Opportunities for Implementing Transformative Learning in Saudi Arabian Higher Education

Implementing transformative learning in Saudi Arabian higher education comes with both challenges and opportunities. While the Vision 2030 plan has set a clear direction towards reform and modernization of the sector, significant efforts must be made to ensure that transformative learning is efficiently used and effectively integrated into the education system in the country.

Cultural norms present a significant challenge to implementing transformative learning in Saudi Arabian higher education. Traditional gender roles and conservative social norms can create resistance to change in higher education settings, especially in mixed-gender classrooms. Therefore, appropriate steps that can overcome these cultural issues must be taken to ensure that the implementation of transformative learning is successful.

Teacher training is crucial for implementing transformative learning in higher education, as educators play a significant role in shaping students' learning experiences. Saudi Arabian universities need to invest in faculty development programs to prepare educators to meet the new demands of teaching and learning techniques. This must include training for different pedagogical strategies and the integration of technology, which would be required for digital transformation. This would help teachers to provide learning with technological training and employ the best fit for various learning styles (Carter et al., 2014).

Another significant challenge is the preparedness of students. Many students in Saudi Arabian higher education institutions come from a background that emphasizes rote memorization and passive engagement with learning. Therefore, the shift towards transformative learning styles that emphasize a problem-based learning approach can be particularly challenging for some students. Educators must work to improve students' critical thinking, problem solving, and collaboration skills to meet the new demands of transformative learning.

Moreover, inadequate infrastructure – technological, classroom, or laboratory – can also create obstacles to harnessing the benefits of transformative learning. There is a need for proper infrastructure to facilitate a student-centred learning experience, for example, virtual labs, online libraries, and a robust digital content repository capable of catering to diverse subjects domains.

There are, of course, many opportunities to implement transformative learning in higher education in Saudi Arabia (Mezirow, 2009). One compelling opportunity is the willingness of the government to invest significantly in improving the education system. The Vision 2030 plan aims to modernize higher education, calling for an increased focus on research, development, and innovation. By focusing on digital transformation and technological developments, higher education institutions in Saudi Arabia can keep pace with innovations in other parts of the world, ensuring that they remain up-to-date and relevant.

Collaboration with international universities is another opportunity for implementing transformative learning in Saudi Arabian higher education. Such partnerships allow for a wealth of knowledge and experience transfer, ultimately enhancing the quality of education provided. Also, developing programs that focus on critical thinking and problem solving, rather than rote memorization, or passive learning, can significantly improve students' overall learning outcomes.

4. Strategies for Implementing Transformative Learning in Saudi Arabian Higher Education

To begin with, transformative learning is a process that involves deep reflection, critical thinking, and the willingness to challenge existing assumptions and beliefs. It involves a shift in perspective that enables learners to develop new insights and skills and to become more self-aware (Eschenbacher & Fleming, 2020; Mezirow, 2009; Percy, 2005; Rojo et al., 2022).

In the context of Saudi Arabian higher education, implementing transformative learning requires a multifaceted approach that involves educators, administrators, and students. Below are some strategies and best practices that can be drawn upon from the global higher education context to implement transformative learning in Saudi Arabian higher education:

1. *Create a supportive learning environment*: A supportive learning environment is essential for facilitating transformative learning. This encompasses creating a learning culture that encourages students to be reflective, ask questions, challenge assumptions, and share their perspectives. Creating a safe and inclusive environment promotes students' willingness to engage in open and honest discussions, leading to transformative learning.
2. *Use technology to enhance learning*: The use of technology is an effective way to engage students and enhance learning experiences. The incorporation of online discussions, video conferencing, and mobile learning platforms can create opportunities for students to collaborate and share content seamlessly. Technology enhances learning by offering numerous resources for educational purposes, such as podcasts, online library resources, e-books, and video tutorials.
3. *Encourage critical thinking and problem solving*: Transformative learning is based on questioning traditional authority and assumptions, engaging with diverse perspectives, and challenging personal beliefs. Therefore, learning experiences should be designed to encourage students to think critically and solve problems through real-life scenarios or case studies.
4. *Promote experiential learning*: Experiential learning is a practice that places the student at the centre of the learning experience. This learning approach emphasizes learning through practice and reflection, ideally in real-world situations. Experiential learning can be offered through internships, apprenticeships, service-learning opportunities, and simulations.
5. *Utilize interdisciplinary approaches*: Interdisciplinary learning involves integrating knowledge and skills from multiple fields. This approach encourages students to think more broadly and develop a deeper understanding of complex problems. In Saudi Arabian higher education, interdisciplinary approaches can be implemented by involving students from various faculties to elaborate on real-world situations.

6. *Foster active learning*: Active learning involves actively engaging students in the learning process, such as by asking questions, participating in group discussions, or collaborating on projects. This approach encourages students to take responsibility for their own learning, which in turn enhances their motivation for learning.

7. *Facilitate continuous self-reflection and assessment*: Transformative learning experiences promote continuous self-reflection and assessment. Learners should have the opportunity to reflect on their progress, evaluate their knowledge, and explore new perspectives. Assessments should also be designed with a focus on feedback and growth rather than solely performance.

In summary, the implementation of transformative learning in Saudi Arabian higher education requires a holistic approach. A supportive learning environment, the use of technology to enhance teaching and learning, encouragement of critical thinking and problem solving, promotion of experiential learning, interdisciplinary approaches, active learning, and continuous self-reflection and assessment are key strategies and best practices. By incorporating these elements, Saudi Arabian higher education can integrate transformative learning and increase learners' knowledge and skills in support of the country's Vision for 2030.

4.1. Pedagogical Approaches for Transformative Learning

In order to facilitate transformative learning in Saudi Arabian higher education, different teaching and learning strategies can be utilized to provide students with the opportunity to engage in critical reflection and challenge their assumptions (Caires-Hurley et al., 2020; Dal Magro et al., 2020; Dunn & Kennedy, 2019; Strange & Gibson, 2017; Thomas, 2009). Three of these strategies are experiential learning, problem-based learning, and technology-enhanced learning. Below is a brief overview of each of these approaches:

1. *Experiential learning*: Experiential learning is a process of learning through experience and reflection. This approach focuses on the idea that knowledge is created through the transformation of experience. It involves activities like field trips, simulations, internships, and service learning that provides students with opportunities to apply theoretical concepts to real-world situations. In Saudi Arabian higher education, experiential learning can be used to facilitate transformative learning by providing students with experiences that provoke reflection and self-discovery through a hands-on approach (Dal Magro et al., 2020; Strange & Gibson, 2017).

2. *Problem-based learning*: Problem-based learning is a student-centred approach that emphasizes the development of critical-thinking skills and the ability to solve complex problems. In this method, students work collaboratively to identify and solve real-world issues. The approach relies on the idea that learning is most effective when it is relevant and engaging. In Saudi Arabian higher education, problem-based learning can be used to facilitate

transformative learning by engaging students in meaningful and collaborative problem-solving experiences (Caires-Hurley et al., 2020).

3. *Technology-enhanced learning*: Technology-enhanced learning involves using technology tools and platforms to facilitate learning. In this approach, technology is used to support learning by providing students with an interactive and engaging experience. Examples of technology-enhanced learning include online chats, mobile learning apps, and virtual reality (VR) environments. In Saudi Arabian higher education, technology-enhanced learning can be used to facilitate transformative learning by providing students with opportunities for self-directed and personalized learning experiences (Dunn & Kennedy, 2019).

In addition to the above teaching and learning approaches, there are other strategies that can also be employed to facilitate transformative learning in Saudi Arabian higher education. These include collaborative learning, case-based learning, and blended learning, among others. The common thread among these approaches is that they all aim to promote active engagement, critical reflection, and the development of conceptual understanding.

There are several teaching and learning strategies that can be utilized to facilitate transformative learning in Saudi Arabian higher education. Experiential learning, problem-based learning, and technology-enhanced learning are three examples of these strategies. Educators can employ a range of tactics to design and facilitate transformative learning experiences for their students, aiming to promote active engagement, critical reflection, and the development of a deep understanding of complex issues.

4.2. Faculty Development for Transformative Learning

Faculty development is essential to foster transformative learning in Saudi Arabian higher education. It is crucial to provide faculty members with the necessary knowledge, skills, and pedagogical approaches to create an environment that supports transformative learning. Below are some recommendations for faculty development programs that can support the implementation of transformative learning in Saudi Arabian higher education:

1. *Training on new pedagogical approaches*: Faculty members need training on new pedagogical approaches to implement transformative learning effectively. This includes training in problem-based learning, experiential learning, reflective practices, and the use of technology-enhanced learning. Faculty members need to be familiar with a range of teaching methods to create a flexible and adaptive learning environment for students.

2. *Cultural competence training*: Cultural competence is crucial for faculty members to understand and respect the diverse cultural backgrounds of students in Saudi Arabian higher education. This includes training in cross-cultural communication, sensitivity, and awareness. Faculty members need to be equipped with intercultural competencies to ensure that teaching and learning align with cultural diversity.

3. *Collaboration and mentoring*: Collaboration and mentoring are key components of faculty development programs. Encouraging interdisciplinary collaboration and mentoring support faculty members to work together and
develop the best practices for teaching and learning. This can also help
bridge the gap between research and teaching in higher education.
4. *Ongoing professional development*: Continuous professional development is
essential for faculty members to keep up with the latest research and methodologies in transformative learning. Ongoing professional development
can take different forms, including attending conferences, workshops, online
courses, and reading and discussing scholarly articles. This is particularly
important because the landscape of higher education is continually changing, and faculty members need to stay up-to-date to provide their students
with the best possible learning experiences.
5. *Student-centred training*: Faculty development programs should be student-
centred, emphasizing the importance of students' needs, goals, and perspectives. This requires training on how to design and implement student-centred
curricula, communicate with students effectively, and encourage critical
thinking and active learning.

Faculty development programs are essential for implementing transformative learning in Saudi Arabian higher education. Training on new pedagogical
approaches, cultural competence, collaboration and mentoring, ongoing professional development, and student-centred training are all necessary components.
Faculty development programs seek to create a culture of constant improvement, aiding and empowering their teaching capacity while accomplishing the
goals of Vision 2030. These programs can help ensure that faculty members are
adequately equipped to foster transformative learning in their students, leading to
positive impacts on Saudi society and the workforce.

4.3. Assessment and Evaluation of Transformative Learning

Assessment and evaluation are vital components of transformative learning in
Saudi Arabian higher education. Assessment and evaluation methods can provide
faculty members and administrators with valuable insights into the effectiveness of
teaching and learning strategies, as well as the impact of transformative learning
on students. Below are some methods for assessing and evaluating transformative
learning outcomes, including student learning, engagement, and satisfaction.

1. *Learning journals and reflective writing*: Learning journals and reflective writing are an effective way to assess and evaluate transformative learning outcomes. Students are asked to write about their learning experiences, focusing
on what they have learned and how their learning has impacted their lives.
Reflective writing enables students to engage in self-reflection, which is a
critical component of transformative learning.
2. *Performance-based assessments*: Performance-based assessments involve
assessing student learning outcomes through measurable tasks or products.

These assessments focus on students' ability to apply what they have learned, rather than solely testing their knowledge retention. For example, students may be asked to apply their knowledge to real-world scenarios or create a project that demonstrates their mastery of a concept or skill.

3. *Surveys and focus groups*: Surveys and focus groups can be used to evaluate student engagement and satisfaction with the learning experience. Surveys can be designed to solicit feedback on specific aspects of the course, such as providing an opportunity for students to discuss their experiences in more depth, providing faculty members with valuable insights into the effectiveness of their teaching and learning strategies.

4. *Peer and self-assessment*: Peer and self-assessment are effective tools for evaluating student learning outcomes. This approach involves having students assess themselves or their peers based on specific criteria. Peer and self-assessment can enhance students' self-awareness and encourage them to take responsibility for their learning.

5. *Rubrics and grading criteria*: Rubrics and grading criteria are tools used to evaluate student performance against specific learning objectives. This approach allows faculty members to provide students with clear feedback on their performance and areas for improvement. Rubrics and grading criteria can also be used to evaluate the effectiveness of teaching and learning strategies.

Assessment and evaluation methods are crucial for evaluating the effectiveness of transformative learning in Saudi Arabian higher education. Methods for assessing and evaluating transformative learning outcomes include learning journals and reflective writing, performance-based assessments, surveys and focus groups, peer and self-assessments, and rubrics and grading criteria. Faculty members and administrators can use these methods to evaluate student learning, engagement, and satisfaction, providing feedback and insight into the effectiveness of their teaching and learning strategies.

5. The Role of Technology in Transformative Learning

In recent years, technology has become an increasingly important tool for facilitating and enhancing transformative learning in higher education institutions in Saudi Arabia. By leveraging the power of technology, educators can create more engaging, interactive, and personalized learning experiences that can help students develop critical-thinking skills and transform the way they think about themselves and the world around them.

One way that technology can facilitate transformative learning is by allowing students to access a wider range of learning resources and experiences than would be possible in traditional classroom settings. With online learning platforms, students can access course materials, lecture recordings, and interactive learning activities from anywhere, at any time. This can help to overcome barriers to learning, such as transportation, scheduling conflicts, or limited access to course materials, and can make it easier for students to engage with course content on their own terms.

Another way that technology can enhance transformative learning is by providing opportunities for collaboration and social learning. Online discussion forums, social media platforms, and virtual learning communities can enable students to connect with each other and with instructors, exchange ideas and perspectives, and foster a sense of community and belonging. This can help to create a more collaborative learning environment, where students can learn from each other and build meaningful relationships that can support their learning and personal growth.

In addition, technology can support more immersive and interactive learning experiences that can help to engage students and promote deeper learning. For example, virtual and augmented reality technologies can be used to create simulations and immersive learning environments that allow students to explore complex concepts and ideas in a more interactive and engaging way. Additionally, gamification strategies, such as incorporating game-like elements, such as points, rewards, and challenges, can help to increase motivation and engagement, making learning more fun and engaging for students.

Finally, technology can be used to personalize learning experiences and provide individualized support to students. With analytics and data-driven insights, educators can track students' progress and identify areas where additional support or interventions may be needed. Adaptive learning technologies can also be used to personalize learning experiences for each student, providing tailored content, feedback, and support based on their individual needs and learning styles.

Technology has the potential to facilitate and enhance transformative learning in Saudi Arabian higher education in many ways. By leveraging the power of technology to create more engaging, interactive, and personalized learning experiences, educators can help students develop critical-thinking skills and transform the way they think about themselves and the world around them. As technology continues to evolve and become more integrated into higher education, we can expect to see even more innovative and transformative uses of technology in the years to come.

5.1. E-Learning and Blended Learning

E-learning and blended learning models have gained popularity in recent years as effective tools for facilitating transformative learning in higher education (Dziuban et al., 2018; Rouleau et al., 2019; Tashkandi, 2021). These models provide a flexible learning environment, allowing students to access educational resources and coursework remotely, while also providing opportunities for interactive collaboration with peers and instructors. While they offer significant benefits, there are also inherent challenges that must be addressed to ensure successful implementation.

One benefit of e-learning and blended learning is the ability to provide students with access to a wide array of educational resources, at any time and from anywhere. This not only saves students time but also allows them to learn at their own pace. Additionally, e-learning and blended learning models allow for more personalized learning environments where content can be adjusted to suit individual students' learning styles and interests. This can help to increase engagement, learning outcomes, and foster transformative learning.

Blended learning models, in particular, have the added advantage of providing opportunities for collaboration and social learning. Through blended learning, students can interact with peers and instructors both online and in-person, which facilitates active participation in the learning process and engagement in online discussions related to course material. This helps students to develop critical-thinking skills while also building valuable relationships that can support their learning and academic success.

Despite their many advantages, e-learning and blended learning models also have inherent challenges that must be addressed. One challenge is ensuring that all students have access to the necessary technology and support to successfully engage with the materials. This issue is particularly acute in areas with limited internet access or technology infrastructure.

Another challenge is ensuring that students remain engaged in the learning process when faced with a lack of face-to-face interactions. Providing structured and interactive online discussions, using multimedia resources, and incorporating student-led group activities can help mitigate disengagement and promote transformative learning.

There are several best practices for integrating technology into the curriculum to ensure that e-learning and blended learning models are effective for transformative learning. One such practice is providing students with adequate support and resources to navigate online learning platforms, resources, and tools. This includes training on the technical aspects of the technology and providing support such as timely and constructive feedback from instructors.

Another best practice is to ensure that the technology used aligns with the student's learning goals, needs, and preferences. The technology should be intuitive, user-friendly, and easy to navigate, as well as complement the course materials and pedagogical goals. Even more so, students should have access to the support material at any time and from any device.

Lastly, it is important to ensure that online interactions in e-learning and blended learning models are related to transformative learning, with a focus on the development of critical-thinking skills, reflective practice, and collaborative problem solving. Pedagogical approaches that involve student-led discussions, problem-based and project-based learning can foster a deeper understanding of course content and its application.

The integration of technology into the curriculum through e-learning and blended learning models can facilitate transformative learning in higher education. While these models offer significant benefits, they are not without challenges that must be addressed. With the right approach to implementation, such as incorporating best practices for technology integration, e-learning, and blended learning models can be an effective tool for transformative learning in the twenty-first century.

5.2. Digital Literacy

Digital literacy are critical components of ensuring that all students have equal access to transformative learning in higher education (Kemp et al., 2021;

O'Doherty et al., 2018). The ability to effectively use technology for learning and communication is becoming increasingly important, however, not all students have equal levels of access to or competencies in technology. It is important to recognize that digital literacy are fundamental components of ensuring that higher education institutions are creating equitable and inclusive learning environments that foster transformative learning.

One way to address the digital divide is through focusing on basic digital literacy skills, such as word processing, email, and internet use. Many higher education institutions offer workshops and training sessions focused on developing these skills or require students to complete introductory digital skills modules before engaging in online coursework. This approach provides individual students with access to basic technological knowledge required for the twenty-first century.

Another way to encourage digital literacy is by incorporating technology into course content through modules and assignments. Educators can work with students to identify technology needs and suggest either free software or low-cost software, and apps to integrate into academic work. This approach can help students develop digital skills and competencies that can be applied to their coursework and connected to real-world applications.

Moreover, to encourage digital literacy and inclusion is by promoting the use of assistive technology that can help to provide all students with equitable learning opportunities. Assistive technology can include voice recognition software, dictation tools, screen magnifiers or readers, and speech-to-text translation software. These technologies can help to level the playing field by allowing students with learning disabilities or poor eyesight to access coursework on an equal footing with their peers.

Finally, higher education institutions should prioritize access to technology and digital literacy for marginalized populations. This can include programs that provide low-cost internet and computer access, or targeted technological training for students from underprivileged backgrounds. It is crucial that all students, regardless of their socioeconomic status, have equal access to digital resources and learning tools.

Digital literacy is crucial components of creating equitable and inclusive learning environments that encourage transformative learning in higher education. By providing training and support for digital literacy, promoting the use of technology in course content and assessments, and prioritizing access for marginalized populations, institutions can ensure that all students can benefit from transformative learning experiences. Furthermore, higher education institutions can also incorporate assistive technology into their curriculum development process to provide digital learning support for students with varied learning styles regardless of their ability levels.

5.3. Emerging Technologies

Emerging technologies have the potential to transform teaching and learning in Saudi Arabian higher education by providing new and innovative ways to engage students, enhance learning experiences, and promote transformative learning outcomes. Here are some examples of emerging technologies that are poised to have a significant impact on higher education in Saudi Arabia (Ho et al., 2020).

VR is one emerging technology that has the potential to transform teaching and learning in higher education. By immersing students in virtual environments, VR can provide a more immersive and engaging learning experience, which can help to foster critical-thinking, problem-solving skills, and creativity. For instance, architects, or civil engineers students, can build, explore, and even spot possible structural design flaws within the virtual world. Medical students can simulate virtual surgeries to get hands-on experience or nursing students can simulate their clinical settings (Bryant et al., 2020; Lie et al., 2023).

Artificial intelligence (AI) is another emerging technology that is poised to revolutionize higher education. By using machine learning algorithms and natural language processing, AI can offer personalized learning experiences that are tailored to each student's strengths and weaknesses, learning styles, and interests. This can help to enhance student engagement and promote transformative learning outcomes by adapting to the student's needs (Yao, 2022).

Gamification is another emerging technology that can be used to promote transformative learning outcomes in higher education. Through the use of game-like elements, such as badges, points, or leaderboards, gamification can increase student motivation and engagement, making learning more fun and interactive. This can help students develop critical-thinking, problem-solving skills, and keep their minds refreshed, thereby supporting transformative learning (Kim & Castelli, 2021).

Augmented reality is an emerging technology that can provide students with an immersive learning experience by integrating digital content with real-world environments. This technology can be used to create interactive learning environments in which students can explore and interact with course materials in new and innovative ways. It also provides learners with practical first-hand information, which they can then apply in real-life situations (Rodríguez-Abad et al., 2021).

These emerging technologies have the potential to promote transformative learning outcomes by providing students with more dynamic and engaging learning experiences. The use of VR, AI, gamification, and augmented reality promotes deep learning outcomes, as opposed to traditional passive learning, as well as hands-on experience, improves productivity, and accelerates cognitive reasoning.

However, integration of these technologies into higher education curricula and pedagogy require careful consideration. Higher education institutions must ensure that these technologies are inclusive and accessible to all students, regardless of their level of technical expertise or access to technology.

Emerging technologies have the potential to transform teaching and learning in higher education in Saudi Arabia by providing more dynamic, immersive, and engaging learning experiences that promote transformative learning outcomes. With careful planning and thoughtful consideration of issues related to accessibility and equity, educators can harness the power of emerging technologies to enhance learning outcomes and prepare students for success in the twenty-first century.

6. Conclusion

This chapter discusses the importance of transformative learning in achieving the Vision 2030 goals for higher education in Saudi Arabia. The authors argue that to prepare students for the complex and changing world, higher education institutions need to move away from traditional teaching methods and adopt transformative learning approaches that encourage critical thinking, reflection, and problem-solving skills. The chapter examines the theoretical foundations of transformative learning, its application in Saudi Arabian higher education, and the challenges associated with its implementation.

We provide several recommendations for future research and practice related to transformative learning in Saudi Arabian higher education. First, they suggest the need for more research on the effectiveness of transformative learning in the Saudi Arabian context. Second, they recommend the development of policies and strategies that promote transformative learning in higher education institutions. Third, they urge the adoption of technology-based approaches that can support transformative learning, such as online learning and VR simulations. Fourth, they emphasize the importance of collaboration between higher education institutions, government agencies, and industry partners to ensure that the knowledge and skills taught align with the needs of the labour market. Finally, they highlight the need for faculty development programs that can equip educators with the necessary knowledge and skills to facilitate transformative learning.

In conclusion, the chapter emphasizes the importance of transformative learning in achieving the Vision 2030 goals for higher education in Saudi Arabia. It provides recommendations for future research and practice related to transformative learning in Saudi Arabian higher education, including more research, policy development, technology adoption, collaboration between stakeholders, and faculty development programs. By adopting transformative learning approaches, higher education institutions in Saudi Arabia can better prepare students for the challenges of the twenty-first century and contribute to the country's economic and social development.

References

Al-Youbi, A. O., Zahed, A. H. M., Nahas, M. N., & Hegazy, A. A. (2021). *The leading world's most innovative universities* (pp. 1–8). Springer Nature.

Al-Hanawi, M. K., Almubark, S., Qattan, A. M., Cenkier, A., & Kosycarz, E. A. (2020). Barriers to the implementation of public-private partnerships in the healthcare sector in the Kingdom of Saudi Arabia. *Plos One, 15*(6), e0233802.

Al-Hanawi, M. K., Khan, S. A., & Al-Borie, H. M. (2019). Healthcare human resource development in Saudi Arabia: Emerging challenges and opportunities – A critical review. *Public Health Review, 40*, 1.

Al-Rabiah Highlights Updates of Transformation Programs and Initiatives 2020 Saudi Ministry of Health. (2019, September 10). https://www.moh.gov.sa/en/Ministry/MediaCenter/News/Pages/News-2019-09-10-003.aspx

Al Bu Ali, W. H., Balaha, M. H., Kaliyadan, F., Bahgat, M., & Aboulmagd, E. (2013). A framework for a competency based medical curriculum in saudi arabia. *Mater Sociomedicine*, *25*(3), 148–152.

Alamri, M. (2011). Higher education in Saudi Arabia. *Journal of Higher Education Theory and Practice*, *11*(4), 88–91.

Alasmari, A. A. (2023). Challenges and social adaptation of international students in Saudi Arabia. *Heliyon*, *9*(5), e16283.

Alebaikan, R., & Troudi, S. (2010). Blended learning in Saudi universities: Challenges and perspectives. *ALT-J, Research in Learning Technology*, *18*(1), 49–59.

Alesawi, A., Malaka, A., Abuzenada, M., Alsaywid, B., Badawood, H., Aldawsari, M., Alshaikh, Y., & Alesawi, N. (2023). Employment rate of newly certified healthcare specialists in Saudi Arabia: A survey-based study. *Cureus*, *15*(6), e40898.

Alfahad, F. N. (2012). Effectiveness of using information technology in higher education in Saudi Arabia. *Procedia-Social and Behavioral Sciences*, *46*, 1268–1278.

Alfawaz, A. A., Salman, K. A., Alotaibi, F. H., Almogbel, F. S., Al-Jaroudi, D., Alrowily, M. J., Derkaoui, A. B., Alqahtani, A. S., Fadlallah, R., Jamal, D., El-Jardali, F., & Memish, Z. A. (2022). Baseline assessment of health research systems in Saudi Arabia: Harnessing efforts and mobilizing actions. *Journal of Epidemiology Global Health*, *12*(4), 400–412.

Alharbi, E. A. R. (2016). Higher education in Saudi Arabia: Challenges to achieving world-class recognition. *International Journal of Culture and History*, *2*(4), 169–172.

Alharbi, H., & Alshammari, M. (2020). Advocacy for democracy in the education system as a part of the Saudi Arabia's Vision 2030. *Journal of Higher Education Theory and Practice*, *20*(8), 129–134.

Alotaibi, N. S. (2022). The significance of digital learning for sustainable development in the Post-COVID19 world in Saudi Arabia's higher education institutions. *Sustainability*, *14*(23), 16219.

Alsanosi, S. M. (2022). A new vision of teaching clinical pharmacology and therapeutics for undergraduate medical students. *Advances in Medical Education and Practice*, *13*, 567–575.

Bataeineh, M., & Aga, O. (2022). Integrating sustainability into higher education curricula: Saudi Vision 2030. *Emerald Open Research*, *4*, 19.

Bin Othayman, M., Mulyata, J., Meshari, A., & Debrah, Y. (2022). The challenges confronting the training needs assessment in Saudi Arabian higher education. *International Journal of Engineering Business Management*, *14*, 18479790211049706.

Bryant, L., Brunner, M., & Hemsley, B. (2020). A review of virtual reality technologies in the field of communication disability: implications for practice and research. *Disability and Rehabilitation: Assistive Technology*, *15*(4), 365–372.

Caires-Hurley, J., Jimenez-Silva, M., & Schepers, O. (2020). Transforming education with problem-based learning: Documenting missed opportunities for multicultural perspectives. *Multicultural Perspectives*, *22*(3), 118–126.

Carter, L., Castano Rodriguez, C., & Jones, M. (2014). Transformative learning in science education: Investigating pedagogy for action. In *Activist science and technology education* (pp. 531–545).

Chowdhury, S., Mok, D., & Leenen, L. (2021). Transformation of health care and the new model of care in Saudi Arabia: Kingdom's Vision 2030. *Journal of Medicine and Life*, *14*(3), 347–354.

Cranton, P. (1994). *Understanding and promoting transformative learning: A guide for educators of adults*. Jossey-Bass.

Dal Magro, R., Pozzebon, M., & Schutel, S. (2020). Enriching the intersection of service and transformative learning with Freirean ideas: The case of a critical experiential learning programme in Brazil. *Management Learning*, *51*(5), 579–597.

Duhaney, D. C. (2005). Technology and higher education: Challenges in the halls of academe. *International Journal of Instructional Media, 32*(1), 7.

Dunn, T. J., & Kennedy, M. (2019). Technology enhanced learning in higher education; Motivations, engagement and academic achievement. *Computers & Education, 137,* 104–113.

Dziuban, C., Graham, C. R., Moskal, P. D., Norberg, A., & Sicilia, N. (2018). Blended learning: The new normal and emerging technologies. *International Journal of Educational Technology in Higher Education, 15*(1), 3.

Eschenbacher, S., & Fleming, T. (2020). Transformative dimensions of lifelong learning: Mezirow, Rorty and COVID-19. *International Review of Education, 66*(5–6), 657–672.

Fisher-Yoshida, B., Geller, K. D., & Schapiro, S. A. (2009). *Innovations in transformative learning: Space, culture, & the arts.* Peter Lang.

Hassounah, M., Raheel, H., & Alhefzi, M. (2020). Digital response during the COVID-19 pandemic in Saudi Arabia. *Journal of Medical Internet Research, 22*(9), e19338.

Ho, D., Quake, S. R., McCabe, E. R. B., Chng, W. J., Chow, E. K., Ding, X., Gelb, B. D., Ginsburg, G. S., Hassenstab, J., Ho, C. M., Mobley, W. C., Nolan, G. P., Rosen, S. T., Tan, P., Yen, Y., & Zarrinpar, A. (2020). Enabling technologies for personalized and precision medicine. *Trends Biotechnology, 38*(5), 497–518.

Kemp, E., Trigg, J., Beatty, L., Christensen, C., Dhillon, H. M., Maeder, A., Williams, P. A. H., & Koczwara, B. (2021). Health literacy, digital health literacy and the implementation of digital health technologies in cancer care: The need for a strategic approach. *Health Promotion Journal of Australia, 32*(Suppl 1), 104–114.

Khalil, R., Mansour, A. E., Fadda, W. A., Almisnid, K., Aldamegh, M., Al-Nafeesah, A., Alkhalifah, A., & Al-Wutayd, O. (2020). The sudden transition to synchronized online learning during the COVID-19 pandemic in Saudi Arabia: a qualitative study exploring medical students' perspectives. *BMC Medical Education, 20*(1), 285.

Kim, J., & Castelli, D. M. (2021). Effects of gamification on behavioral change in education: A meta-analysis. *International Journal of Environmental Research and Public Health, 18*(7), 3550.

Lie, S. S., Helle, N., Sletteland, N. V., Vikman, M. D., & Bonsaksen, T. (2023). Implementation of virtual reality in health professions education: Scoping review. *JMIR Medical Education, 9,* e41589.

Magkoufopoulou, C. (2023). The role of active learning in transformative learning and teaching experiences. In W. Garnham & I. Gowers (Eds.), *Active learning in higher education* (pp. 34–45). Routledge.

Mezirow, J. (2009). Transformative learning theory. In J. Mezirow & E. W. Taylor (Eds.), *Transformative learning in practice: Insights from community, workplace, and higher education* (pp. 18–31). Jossey-Bass.

Mitchell, B., & Alfuraih, A. (2018). The Kingdom of Saudi Arabia: Achieving the aspirations of the National Transformation Program 2020 and Saudi vision 2030 through education. *Journal of Education and Development, 2*(3), 36.

Mohiuddin, K., Nasr, O. A., Nadhmi Miladi, M., Fatima, H., Shahwar, S., Noorulhasan Naveed, Q. (2023). Potentialities and priorities for higher educational development in Saudi Arabia for the next decade: Critical reflections of the vision 2030 framework. *Heliyon, 9*(5), e16368.

Nurunnabi, M. (2017). Transformation from an oil-based economy to a knowledge-based economy in Saudi Arabia: The direction of Saudi vision 2030. *Journal of the Knowledge Economy, 8,* 536–564.

O'Doherty, D., Dromey, M., Lougheed, J., Hannigan, A., Last, J., & McGrath, D. (2018). Barriers and solutions to online learning in medical education – An integrative review. *BMC Medical Education, 18*(1), 130.

Percy, R. (2005). The contribution of transformative learning theory to the practice of participatory research and extension: Theoretical reflections. *Agriculture and Human Values, 22,* 127–136.

Reay, S., & Collier, G. (2017). Designing situated learning experiences: Interdisciplinary collaboration for design education in healthcare. *Studies in Health Technology and Informatics, 242*, 1030–1033.

Rodríguez-Abad, C., Fernández-de-la-Iglesia, J. D., Martínez-Santos, A. E., & Rodríguez-González, R. (2021). A systematic review of augmented reality in health sciences: A guide to decision-making in higher education. *International Journal of Environmental Research and Public Health, 18*(8), 4262.

Rojo, J., Ramjan, L., George, A., Hunt, L., Heaton, L., Kaur, A., & Salamonson, Y. (2022). Applying Mezirow's transformative learning theory into nursing and health professional education programs: A scoping review. *Teaching and Learning in Nursing, 18*(1), 63–71.

Rouleau, G., Gagnon, M. P., Côté, J., Payne-Gagnon, J., Hudson, E., Dubois, C. A., & Bouix-Picasso, J. (2019). Effects of e-learning in a continuing education context on nursing care: Systematic review of systematic qualitative, quantitative, and mixed-studies reviews. *Journal of Medical Internet Research, 21*(10), e15118.

Saudi Vision 2030 An ambitious vision for an ambitious nation. (2023). [cited 2023 March 10]. https://www.vision2030.gov.sa

Shahwan, R., & Zaman, T. (2023). Role of universities as knowledge creators in a national innovation system: An open innovation paradigm. In *Industry clusters and innovation in the Arab world: Challenges and opportunities* (pp. 259–280). Emerald Publishing Limited.

Smart Government Strategy in the Kingdom of Saudi Arabia my.gov.sa. https://www.my.gov.sa/wps/portal/snp/aboutksa/smartstrategy/?lang=en

Smith, L., & Abouammoh, A. (2013). *Higher education in Saudi Arabia: Reforms, challenges and priorities* (pp. 1–12). Springer.

Strange, H., & Gibson, H. J. (2017). An investigation of experiential and transformative learning in study abroad programs. *Frontiers: The Interdisciplinary Journal of Study Abroad, 29*(1), 85–100.

Strecker, S., Kundisch, D., Lehner, F., Leimeister, J. M., & Schubert, P. (2018). Higher education and the opportunities and challenges of educational technology. *Business & Information Systems Engineering, 60*, 181–189.

Tashkandi, E. (2021). E-learning for undergraduate medical students. *Advances in Medical Education and Practice, 12*, 665–674.

Taylor, E. W., & Tisdell, E. J. (2017). Patricia Cranton and transformative learning theory: An integrated perspective. *Adult Education Quarterly, 54*(4), 1–10.

Thomas, I. (2009). Critical thinking, transformative learning, sustainable education, and problem-based learning in universities. *Journal of Transformative Education, 7*(3), 245–264.

Thompson, M. C. (2017). 'Saudi vision 2030': A viable response to youth aspirations and concerns? *Asian Affairs, 48*(2), 205–221.

Uddin, M., & Alharbi, N. K. (2023). The landscape of biomedical research progress, challenges and prospects in Saudi Arabia – A systematic review. *Digital Health, 9*, 20552076231178621

Vipler, B., Knehans, A., Rausa, D., Haidet, P., & McCall-Hosenfeld, J. (2021). Transformative learning in graduate medical education: A scoping review. *The Journal of Graduate Medical Education, 13*(6), 801–814.

Vipler, B., Snyder, B., McCall-Hosenfeld, J., Haidet, P., Peyrot, M., & Stuckey, H. (2022). Transformative learning of medical trainees during the COVID-19 pandemic: A mixed methods study. *PLoS One, 17*(9), e0274683.

Yao, G. (2022). Application of higher education management in colleges and universities by deep learning. *Computational Intelligence and Neuroscience, 2022*, 7295198.

Printed and bound by CPI Group (UK) Ltd, Croydon, CR0 4YY

20/11/2023

08191577-0001